The Slimming Foodie AIR FRYER

hamlyn

First published in Great Britain in 2025 by Hamlyn, an imprint of
Octopus Publishing Group Ltd
Carmelite House
50 Victoria Embankment
London EC4Y 0DZ
www.octopusbooks.co.uk
An Hachette UK Company
www.hachette.co.uk

The authorized representative in the EEA is Hachette Ireland, 8 Castlecourt Centre,
Dublin 15, D15 XTP3, Ireland (email: info@hbgi.ie)

Text copyright © Pip Payne 2025
Photography copyright © Chris Terry 2025
Design and layout copyright © Octopus Publishing Group Ltd 2025

Distributed in the US by Hachette Book Group
1290 Avenue of the Americas, 4th and 5th Floors
New York, NY 10104

Distributed in Canada by Canadian Manda Group
664 Annette St., Toronto, Ontario, Canada M6S 2C8

ISBN 978 0 60063 898 8

A CIP catalogue record for this book is available from the British Library.
Printed and bound in Italy.

10 9 8 7 6 5 4 3 2 1

Publisher: Kate Fox
Editorial Director: Natalie Bradley
Senior Managing Editor: Sybella Stephens
Copy Editor: Lucy Bannell
Art Director: Yasia Williams
Photographer: Chris Terry
Food Stylist: Henrietta Clancy
Props Stylist: Tamsin Weston
Production Controllers: Lucy Carter & Nic Jones

The Slimming Foodie AIR FRYER

Quick, easy, healthy meals all under 600 calories

PIP PAYNE

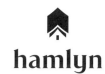

hamlyn

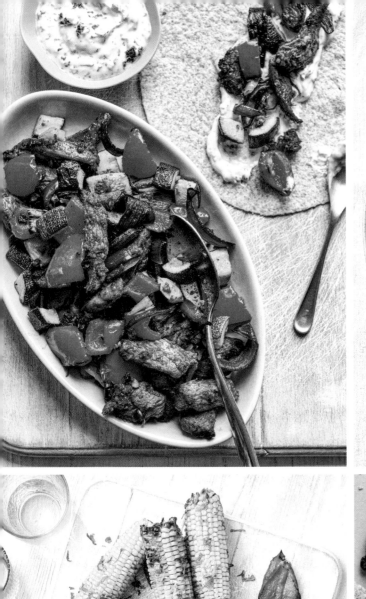
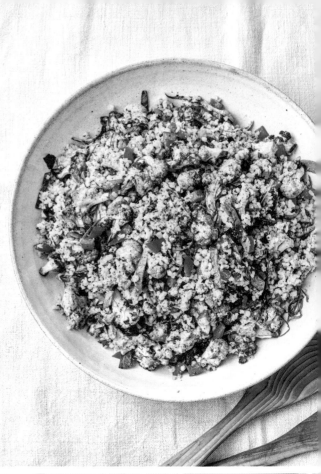
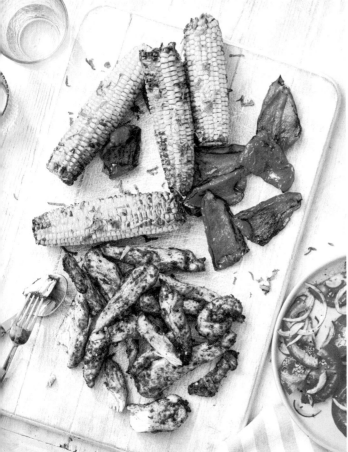
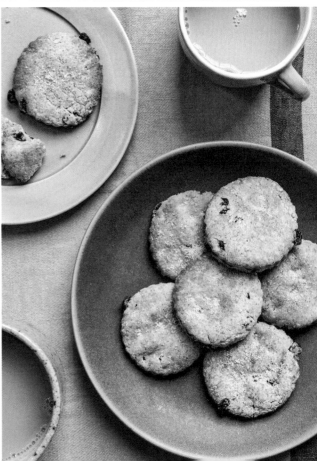

Contents

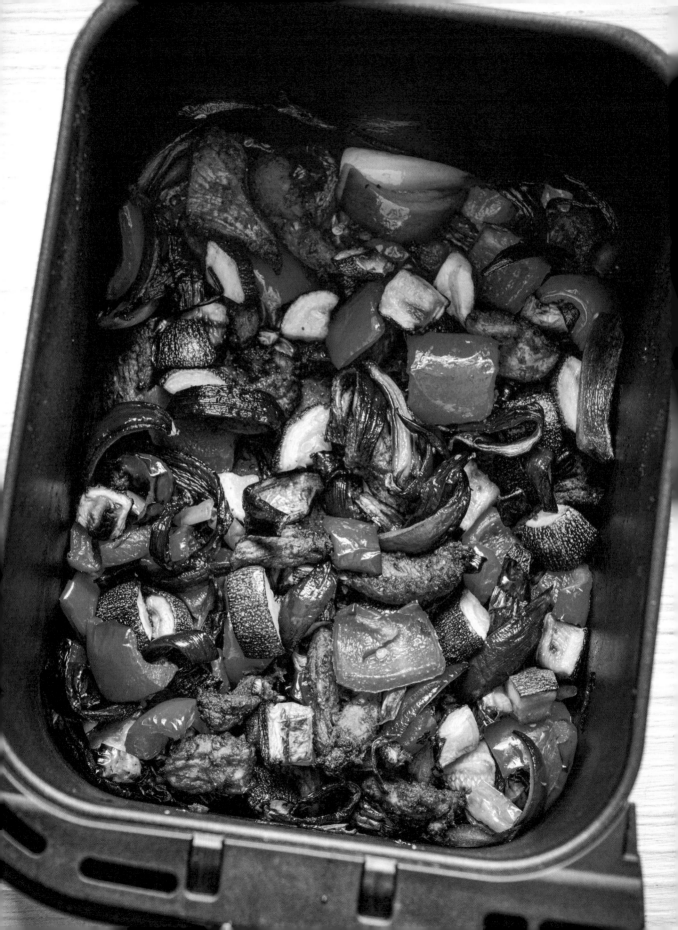

INTRODUCTION

Air fryers have exploded! They are now an essential piece of kitchen kit, so it made sense to add an air fryer cookbook to The Slimming Foodie collection; recipes for air fryers have certainly been among the most-requested by my online community over recent months.

This book is for anyone looking to make healthy, wholesome home-cooked meals in their air fryer, whether you are a newbie or a seasoned pro. From quick and easy snacks to hearty family favourites and delicious desserts, the recipes in these pages offer something for every occasion.

Air fryers speed up cooking times and add a level of versatility to your kitchen, as they are a cost-effective alternative to a traditional oven. They were originally thought of as a healthier alternative to a frying pan (hence the name), allowing you to enjoy crisp, delicious meals made with less oil. But air fryers aren't only good for crispy food – you can use them to cook a huge range of dishes. I have tried to put as many types of recipes as I can into this book to show you what your air fryer can do, from soup to pasta to curry, there really is so much to discover.

WHICH AIR FRYER?

Of course, there are so many different models and makes of air fryer out there that it's impossible to accommodate every type into a single book. For the recipes here, I have used a dual-drawer model with a 7.6–9.5-litre (8–10 quart) capacity. This is the type of air fryer that I most commonly see used, and that these recipes have been tested in. As with all my other books, I wanted most of the meals to serve four people, for which this type of air fryer is perfect, as you can cook two separate elements at once. However, even if you have a single-drawer air fryer, you'll find most of my recipes very easy to adapt to suit it.

HANDS-ON AIR FRYING

One of my first realizations with a drawer-based air fryer is that it's not a hands-off process, as it used to be with older models which had a turning paddle. You do need to attend to the food – turning, shaking or checking. But don't worry: for many of the dishes in this book, you can be preparing other elements of a meal while the air fryer is doing its thing, and the machines are so efficient that you won't be stuck in the kitchen for hours on end.

REAL-LIFE COOKING

In this book, you'll see that I've used a hob to cook certain elements of a meal, as I think this reflects how we actually cook; I generally use a combination of my air fryer and hob to create my family's meals, so that's what I've done here too. Of course, there are some meals you can cook solely in the air fryer, but I have based my recipes on how I cook day-to-day. With ingredients such as rice, I know you can buy pouches of microwaveable grains, but they are expensive and create unnecessary waste; to me, it makes much more sense just to cook the rice on the hob.

EQUIPMENT & ACCESSORIES

I have tried to limit the use of items such as baking dishes to make the meals for this book. It's hard to recommend specific-sized dishes because there is so much variation, and this can have a big effect on cooking time, so most of these recipes are made directly in the air fryer drawers, with or without the crisper plates fitted. You may yourself use silicone drawer liners, and I do occasionally, but I prefer cooking directly in the drawer as I think it gives the best results. Where needed, I have used a few simple containers in the recipes, such as ramekins and silicone cupcake cases, which are very easily available.

IMPORTANT TIPS

Please read this before embarking on the recipes!

- Having tested these recipes using a variety of air fryers and different models, I can confirm that each cooks very differently, even when set to the same temperature. If you've had your air fryer for a while, you have probably already worked out how it cooks and how to adjust recipes to suit it, but if you have a new machine, it can take a little bit of getting used to. Because of this, the timings and temperatures in this book should be taken as a general guide. You may need to adapt your approach to the recipes depending on your model of air fryer. If you notice that food seems to be burning on top when it still has a significant time left to cook (especially meat), it's advisable to reduce the temperature, or cover the food with foil to prevent further scorching. Conversely, if something isn't browning as much as it should, you can increase the temperature or the cooking time. Different air fryers have various settings, but for this book the recipes were all tested on 'air fry' mode.

- Air fryers tend to be very good at making things look cooked on the outside, so I highly recommend investing in a meat thermometer; they are not expensive and knowing that your meat is safely cooked all the way through can give you peace of mind. The manufacturer's instructions will tell you what temperature is safe for which type of meat.

- Take meat out of the fridge 30–60 minutes before cooking. Fridge-cold meat can make a significant difference to the timing of recipes, as it will often overcook on the outside before it is cooked through to the middle.

- I recommend preheating your air fryer. It only takes a few minutes and it can give you a more evenly cooked result, as well as making sure that the timings for the recipes work as they should.

- **Never line the air fryer drawers before preheating.** For any recipes that use baking paper or foil, only add it – weighted down with the food – after the air fryer has preheated. If the sheet of paper or foil is not securely weighted down by food, it will blow around and can catch fire on the heating element, which can obviously be dangerous.

- Unless stated in the recipes, the crisper plates (or grill trays) should be left inside the air fryer drawers during cooking.

- Please make sure you have read the manufacturer's instructions for your own air fryer. There are quirks to different models, and it's important that you understand your own machine, as well as the recommended cleaning methods. Personally, I do not put my air fryer drawers or crisper plates in the dishwasher, as it is likely to reduce the lifespan of the nonstick coating. They are very easy to clean with a quick wash by hand after every use.

- Most air fryers that I have used recommend avoiding low-calorie cooking spray to ensure the lifespan of the nonstick coating, so I most often use a refillable food-grade spray bottle (easy to find online and not expensive), filled with olive oil. You will find that some of these recipes use a specified amount of oil, because I have found the results are much better. In most cases, for a meal serving four people, the amount of oil is negligible and adds only a few calories. I think it's fully worth embracing this approach for the overall result, because all the recipes are for good, home-cooked food that beats any ready meal.

AIR FRYING EQUIPMENT

My most-used kitchen tools with an air fryer are:
- Silicone tongs
- Silicone spoon or spatula
- Silicone pastry brush
- Oil spray bottle
- Meat thermometer
- Nonstick baking paper
- Metal skewers (20cm / 8 inches)
- Silicone cupcake cases
- Ramekins
- Medium-sized takeaway foil trays

ONLINE COMMUNITY

Please feel free to head over to The Slimming Foodie Facebook page and join in our community, where we share air fryer tips, recipes, inspiration and successes. And don't forget to tag me on social media when you have made one of my recipes, as I love to see my books come to life!

www.theslimmingfoodie.com

slimmingfoodie

the_slimming_foodie

GENERAL NOTES

- **Prep and cook times:** I give estimates for the time it takes to chop, grate or mix. I'm not an expert chopper, so I'd say that these timings are for an intermediate home cook. If cooking is new to you, it may take you a little longer.

- Generally, I choose **fresh garlic** or **ginger** rather than tubes or jars of prepared pastes, as I think the taste is better and because there are no preservatives. But if you are really in a rush, there's no harm in using a convenient paste.

- I often specify **'coarsely ground salt'**, which just means I'm not using fine table salt, as a teaspoon of that will give a different level of salty taste.

- All **eggs** are large and free-range.

- All **butter** is salted, unless otherwise stated.

- **Get organized.** There are two secrets to a successful meal: first, prep your ingredients in advance, and second, quickly read through the full recipe to make sure there aren't any surprises!

- The **calorie counts** in the meals are for a single portion and do not include serving suggestions or side dishes that aren't listed with the other ingredients. Occasionally, I'll add a side dish to a recipe, so I include it in the calorie count, but most of the time I'll leave it for you to decide what works best.

- **Portion sizes** are difficult to estimate, as a family with two toddlers will need a very different amount of food from a family with two teenagers! I base my portion sizes on recommended amounts, as well as my experience of making the dish and what I consider to be a satisfying portion. Of course, this is subjective, so you may need to adjust the portions to work for you and your family. Just please be aware that the air fryer timings will not work if you overfill the machine, and that you may need to cook food in batches if you are making a larger amount. It's always worth cooking extra vegetables on the side for filling-power, if you think you might need them. I also realize that not every family or household is made up of four people, so you will find that many of the recipes are easy to scale up or down, or you could make the full amount and freeze any leftover portions for another day.

- I make suggestions for **freezer-friendly** food based on what I consider gives good results when defrosted. You may well be able to freeze meals not marked as freezer-friendly, but their consistency may suffer once reheated. Always allow food to cool fully before placing in the freezer. Transfer leftovers to airtight plastic containers or freezer bags, then label them with the contents and date. Make sure food is thoroughly defrosted before reheating.

- All recipes are designed to be lower in fat and calories, but I know that many people who enjoy cooking from my books are not watching either of those. Please feel free to use the full-fat version of any ingredients, such as sausages, coconut milk or cream cheese, as these will only make the meals taste even better... and I love the fact that my recipes are enjoyed by all!

SYMBOLS

Look out for these symbols at the top of each recipe:

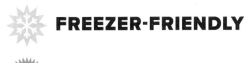

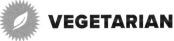

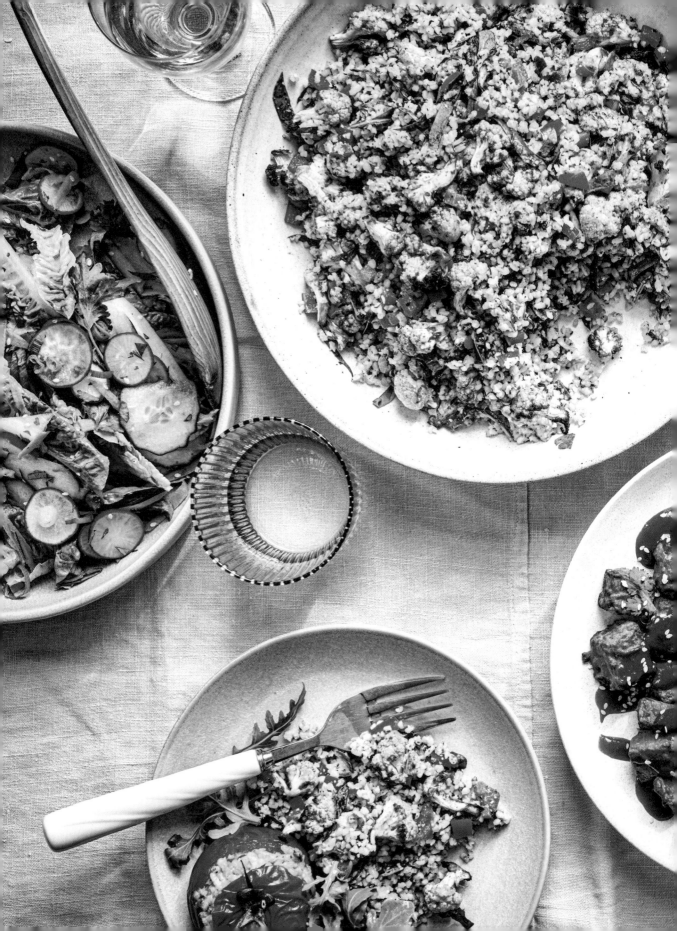

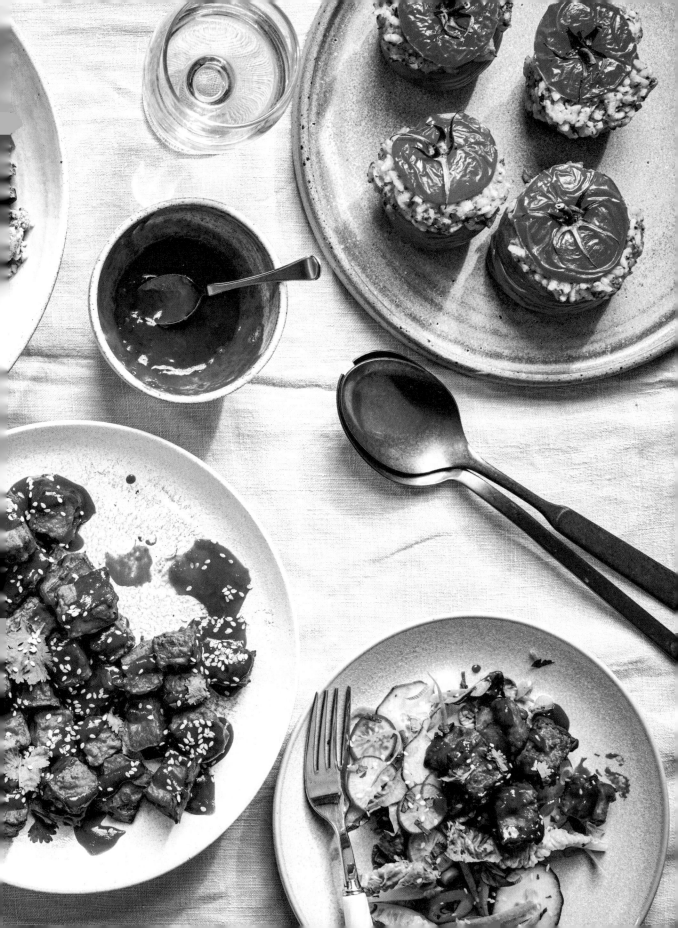

BLUEBERRY, ALMOND &
CINNAMON BAKED OATS

HONEY CRUNCH GRANOLA

SESAME & SULTANA
FLATBREADS

BANANA PUFF PANCAKES

STEM GINGER & PECAN
GRANOLA

CHERRY BAKEWELL BAGELS

TOP HAT CRISPY POTATO
SKINS

SWEET CHILLI MUSHROOMS
& POACHED EGG ON TOAST

1

Breakfast & brunch

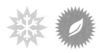

BLUEBERRY, ALMOND & CINNAMON BAKED OATS

SERVES 2
PREP TIME 5 minutes
COOK TIME 12 minutes

---

spray oil

80g porridge oats (not jumbo oats)

2 tablespoons ground almonds

2 teaspoons baking powder

1 teaspoon ground cinnamon

1 egg, lightly beaten

4 tablespoons fat-free Greek yogurt, plus more to serve

1 tablespoon maple syrup, or honey, or golden syrup

1 teaspoon vanilla extract

100g fresh blueberries (please note frozen blueberries will affect the cooking time)

This has (quite rightly) always been one of the most popular recipes on The Slimming Foodie blog, and it's fantastic baked in the air fryer. I make up single portions in ramekins, though it's easy to scale up this recipe if you want to make a bigger batch in one go because it reheats well. You don't have to add ground almonds, but for me they really add an extra dimension to the taste. I serve this with more Greek yogurt and fresh berries, such as blueberries, raspberries and strawberries.

1 Preheat 1 air fryer drawer to 180°C (350°F). Spray 2 ramekins with oil.

2 Mix together the oats, ground almonds, baking powder and cinnamon, then add the egg, yogurt, maple syrup and vanilla extract and stir well to combine all the ingredients. Stir through the blueberries, then divide the mixture between the ramekins.

3 Put the ramekins in the air fryer drawer and cook for 8–12 minutes. Check them after 6 minutes – in some air fryers the tops will brown more quickly than others, in which case cover the ramekins securely with foil to prevent the tops from overcooking.

4 To check that they are cooked through (cooking times can vary slightly depending on your air fryer), insert a butter knife into the middle of a ramekin: the baked oats should be cake-like and not still sloppy in the middle. If they need more time, continue to cook in 2-minute increments, checking on them after each.

PER SERVING

CALORIES	FAT	SAT FAT	CARBS	SUGARS	FIBRE	PROTEIN	SALT
354	12G	1.2G	40G	13G	6G	17G	1.6G

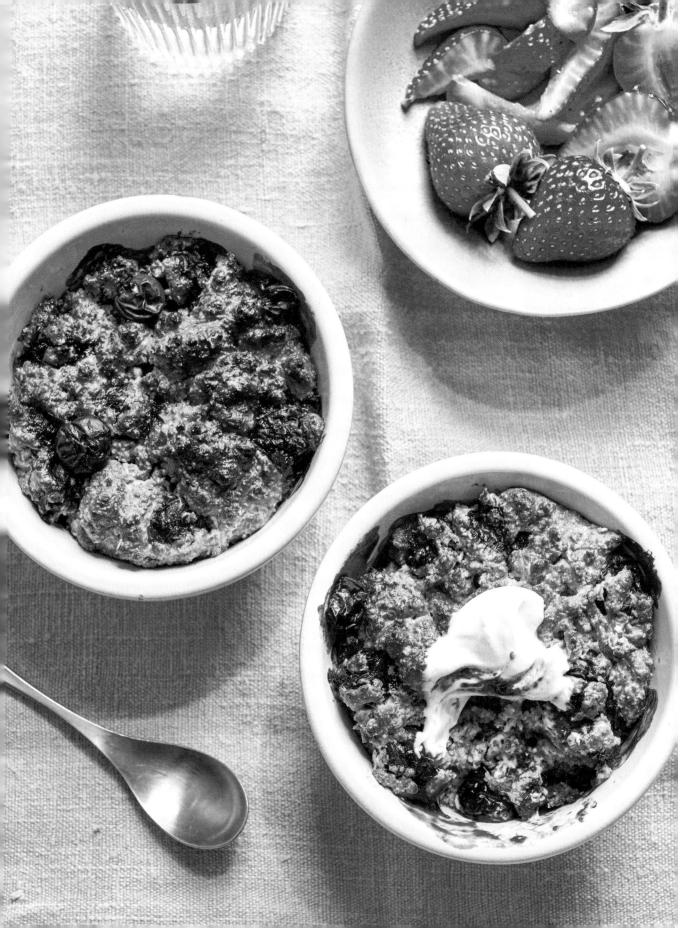

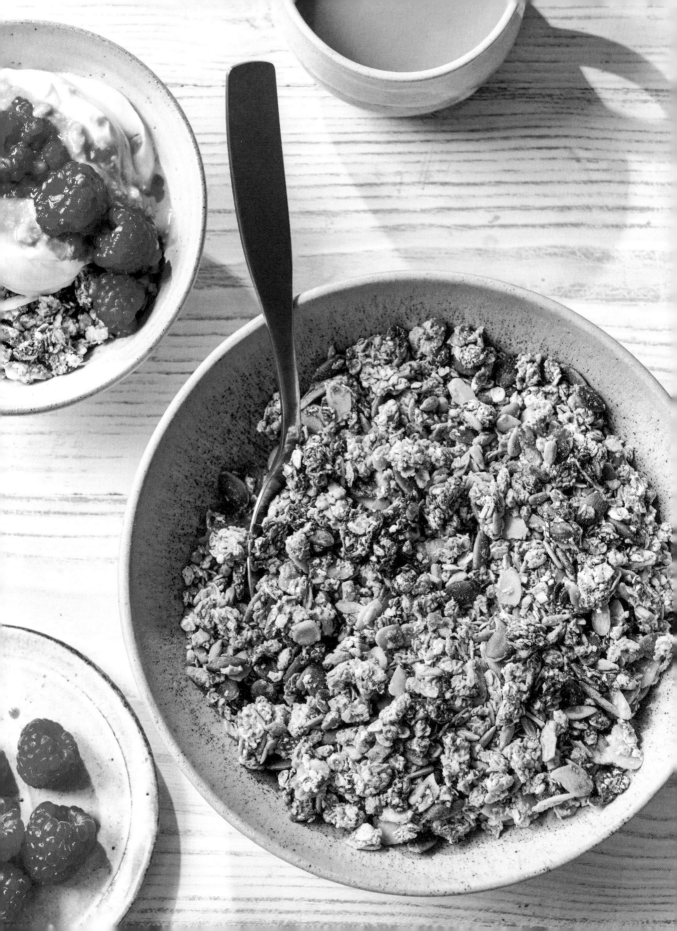

HONEY CRUNCH GRANOLA

MAKES 8 portions
PREP TIME 5 minutes
COOK TIME 15–18 minutes

160g (5¾oz) porridge oats
 (not jumbo oats)
40g (1½oz) sunflower seeds
40g (1½oz) pumpkin seeds
30g (1oz) flaked almonds
1 egg
2 tablespoons honey
1 teaspoon vanilla extract

Granola is my everyday breakfast. This delicious, crunchy version makes the perfect start to a day when served with Greek yogurt and fresh berries. I also love a teaspoon of crunchy peanut butter with my portion. I use egg in this granola to help the flavours really coat the oats and seeds, creating that great crunch, as well as some clusters.

1 Preheat both air fryer drawers to 175°C (345°F).

2 Put the oats in a mixing bowl with the sunflower seeds, pumpkin seeds and flaked almonds. In another bowl, whisk together the egg, honey and vanilla extract. Pour the egg mixture into the oat mixture, then stir thoroughly to mix and coat everything with the egg mixture.

3 Carefully line the hot air fryer drawers with nonstick baking paper or silicone liners, then spoon half the granola mixture into each drawer in an even layer. Cook for 15 minutes, stirring it every 5 minutes. You want to make sure that the crisp bits on the top and around the sides are mixed in, and that bigger clumps are broken up every time, to make sure it all has a chance to crisp.

4 After 15 minutes, stir it again. If you feel that there is still a little bit of dampness in it, then pop it back into the air fryer for a few more minutes to cook a little bit more. Once it's done, it should be golden and crisp.

5 Remove the air fryer drawers and place on a heatproof surface to allow the granola to steam off and completely cool. (Don't leave it in a closed drawer, as the remaining steam may cause it to go soft.)

6 Once it is completely cool, you can transfer it into a glass jar or airtight container, where it will keep for up to 10 days.

PER SERVING

CALORIES	FAT	SAT FAT	CARBS	SUGARS	FIBRE	PROTEIN	SALT
156	8.4G	1.2G	13G	3.8G	2.2G	5.4G	TRACE

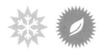

SESAME & SULTANA FLATBREADS

MAKES 8
PREP TIME 5 minutes
COOK TIME 12 minutes

250g (9oz) self-raising flour, plus more to dust

1 teaspoon baking powder

2 teaspoons ground cinnamon

250g (9oz) fat-free Greek yogurt

40g (1½oz) sesame seeds

40g (1½oz) sultanas

salt

These are chewy and delicious and remind me of bagels, both the cinnamon-raisin and sesame varieties combined! They are lovely hot, straight from the air fryer, spread with butter or low-fat spread and honey, or just as delicious cold on their own.

1   Mix the flour, baking powder and cinnamon thoroughly in a bowl before adding the rest of the ingredients and a pinch of salt. Bring the dough together in the bowl, kneading until it becomes a single ball.

2   Using floured hands, divide the dough into 8 balls, then stretch each piece into a roundish 8cm (3¼ inch) flatbread. Make sure 2 will fit comfortably in each air fryer drawer.

3   Preheat both air fryer drawers to 180°C (350°F).

4   Place 2 flatbreads in each drawer and cook for 6 minutes, flipping once during cooking. Repeat to cook the remaining 4 flatbreads.

PER FLATBREAD

CALORIES	FAT	SAT FAT	CARBS	SUGARS	FIBRE	PROTEIN	SALT
174	3.4G	0.7G	27G	4.6G	2.4G	7.3G	0.51G

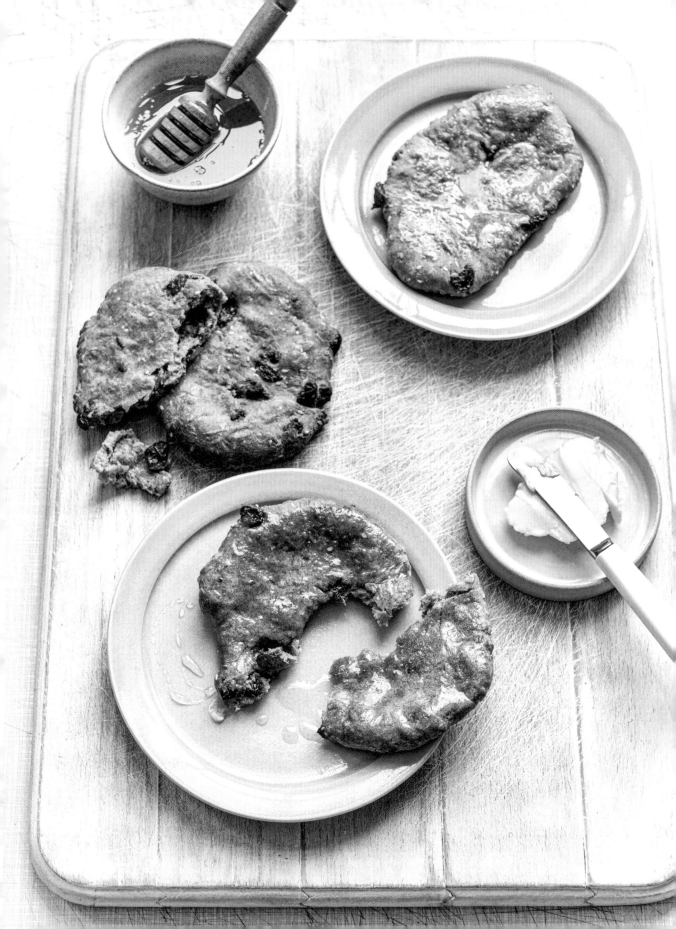

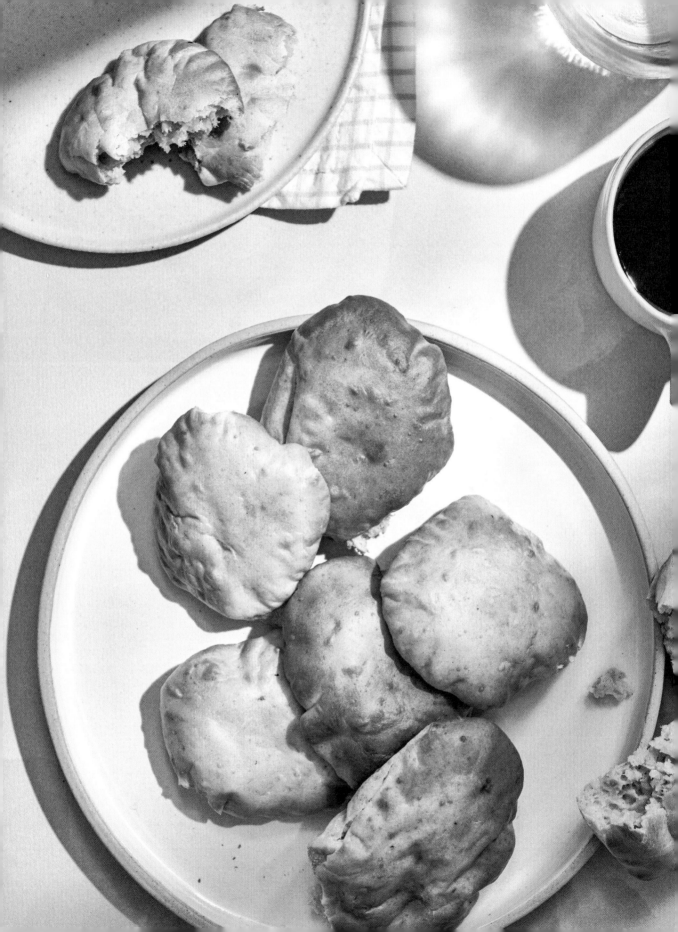

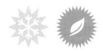

BANANA PUFF PANCAKES

MAKES 8
PREP TIME 5 minutes
COOK TIME 8 minutes

1 ripe banana
1 egg, lightly beaten
1 tablespoon fat-free Greek yogurt
70ml (2½fl oz) milk
1 teaspoon vanilla extract
170g (6oz) self-raising flour
couple of gratings of nutmeg

Somewhere between a fluffy pancake and a little cake, these are delicious as they are, sliced open and used like a cheat's brioche, or topped with a dollop of yogurt. They are usually sweet enough, despite containing no sugar, but if your banana isn't perfectly ripe, you can add a teaspoon of honey or maple syrup to the batter.

1   Start by squishing the peeled banana on a plate with a fork until it turns into a paste. Transfer to a bowl and add the egg, yogurt, milk and vanilla and whisk thoroughly until combined.

2   In a separate bowl, whisk the flour and nutmeg together.

3   Mix the wet ingredients into the dry until you have a lump-free batter.

4   Preheat both air fryer drawers to 160°C (325°F).

5   Carefully line both hot drawers with nonstick baking paper, then use a tablespoon to spoon 4 pancakes into each drawer: it doesn't matter if they touch each other a little. Cook for 8 minutes, turning halfway through. They should be puffed up and golden when they are ready.

PER PANCAKE

CALORIES	FAT	SAT FAT	CARBS	SUGARS	FIBRE	PROTEIN	SALT
191	2.2G	0.7G	34G	5.4G	1.9G	7G	0.41G

STEM GINGER & PECAN GRANOLA

MAKES 8 portions
PREP TIME 5 minutes
COOK TIME 15 minutes

120g (4¼oz) jumbo oats

80g (2¾oz) pecan nuts, roughly chopped

60g (2¼oz) sunflower seeds

40g (1½oz) crystallized ginger, finely chopped

2 tablespoons maple syrup

1 teaspoon olive oil

1 tablespoon orange juice

coarsely ground salt

A lovely blend of warm spices and crunchy textures, perfect for a wholesome breakfast or brunch. Easy to prepare in an air fryer, the crystallized ginger and rich pecans give this granola a unique flavour. This is delicious served with yogurt and fresh fruit such as sliced apples or pears.

1 Mix the dry ingredients in a large bowl with a pinch of salt.

2 Whisk the wet ingredients together in a separate bowl, then pour them into the oat mixture and mix thoroughly.

3 Preheat both air fryer drawers to 150°C (300°F).

4 Carefully line the hot air fryer drawers with nonstick baking paper or silicone liners, then spoon half the granola into each drawer in an even layer. Cook for 15 minutes, stirring every 5 minutes to ensure even cooking.

5 After 15 minutes, stir it again. If you feel that there is still a little dampness in it, pop it back into the air fryer for a few more minutes to cook it a little bit more. Once it's done, it should be golden and crisp.

6 Remove the air fryer drawers and place on a heatproof surface to allow the granola to steam off and completely cool in the drawers. (Don't leave it in a closed drawer, as the remaining steam may cause it to go soft.)

7 Once the granola is completely cool, you can transfer it into a glass jar or airtight container, where it will keep for up to 10 days.

PER SERVING

CALORIES	FAT:	SAT FAT	CARBS	SUGARS	FIBRE	PROTEIN	SALT
198	12G	1.4G	16G	5.7G	3G	4.3G	TRACE

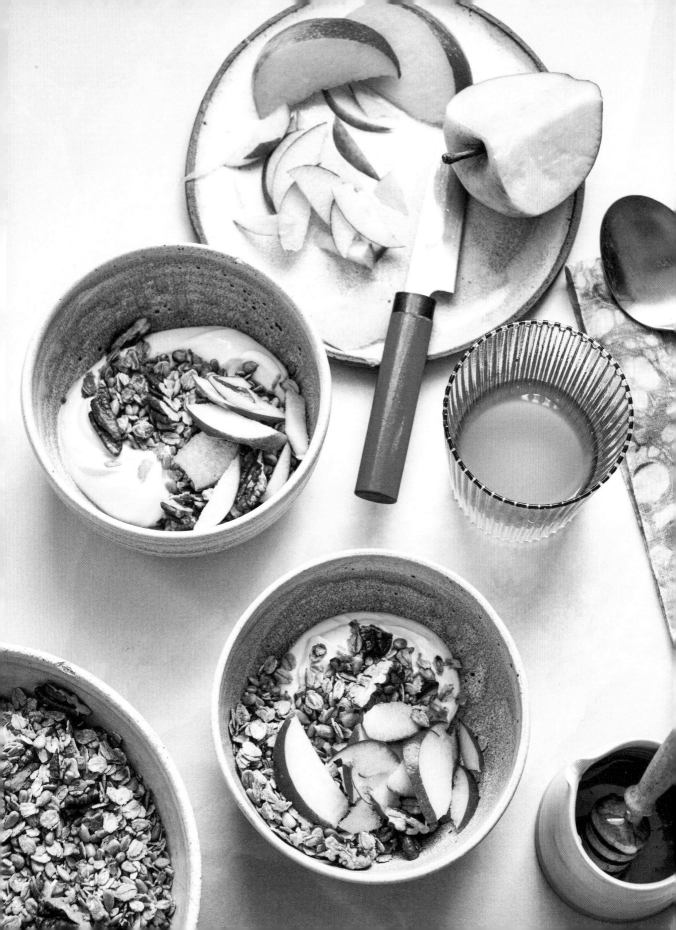

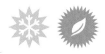

CHERRY BAKEWELL BAGELS

MAKES 4
PREP TIME 20 minutes
COOK TIME 12 minutes

Sweet roasted cherries and almonds are a perfect pairing in a warm and doughy bagel. A little almond crunch on top finishes them off. These can be eaten just as they are, or served with butter or jam.

160g (5¾oz) self-raising flour, plus more if needed and to dust

130g (4¾oz) fat-free Greek yogurt

120g (4¼oz) fresh pitted cherries, or frozen and defrosted cherries, finely chopped

1 tablespoon honey

1 teaspoon almond extract

10g (¼oz) flaked almonds

1 egg, lightly beaten

1 Place the flour and yogurt in a mixing bowl and use a fork to combine them and start to form a dough. Add the cherries, honey and almond extract, using the fork to combine them, then use your hands to form the dough into a ball. Please note that different brands of yogurt can affect the texture, so if the dough is too sticky, add a little more flour until you are able to handle it.

2 Divide the dough into 4 equal pieces and use floured hands and a floured work surface to roll each piece into a long sausage shape, around 20cm (8 inches) in length. Form each sausage into a bagel by connecting the 2 ends, then using your fingers to press and squeeze the dough until it has sealed together and formed a nice round bagel with a hole in the middle. Press the flaked almonds gently on to the tops, dividing them equally between the 4 bagels.

3 Using a silicone pastry brush, gently brush each bagel with beaten egg, trying not to dislodge the almonds.

4 Preheat both air fryer drawers to 180°C (350°F).

5 Place 2 bagels in each air fryer drawer and cook for 12 minutes. Check on them after 10 minutes to ensure that the almonds on top aren't getting overcooked.

PER BAGEL

CALORIES	FAT	SAT FAT	CARBS	SUGARS	FIBRE:	PROTEIN	SALT
229	3.4G	0.7G	38G	8.6G	2.5G	9G	0.44G

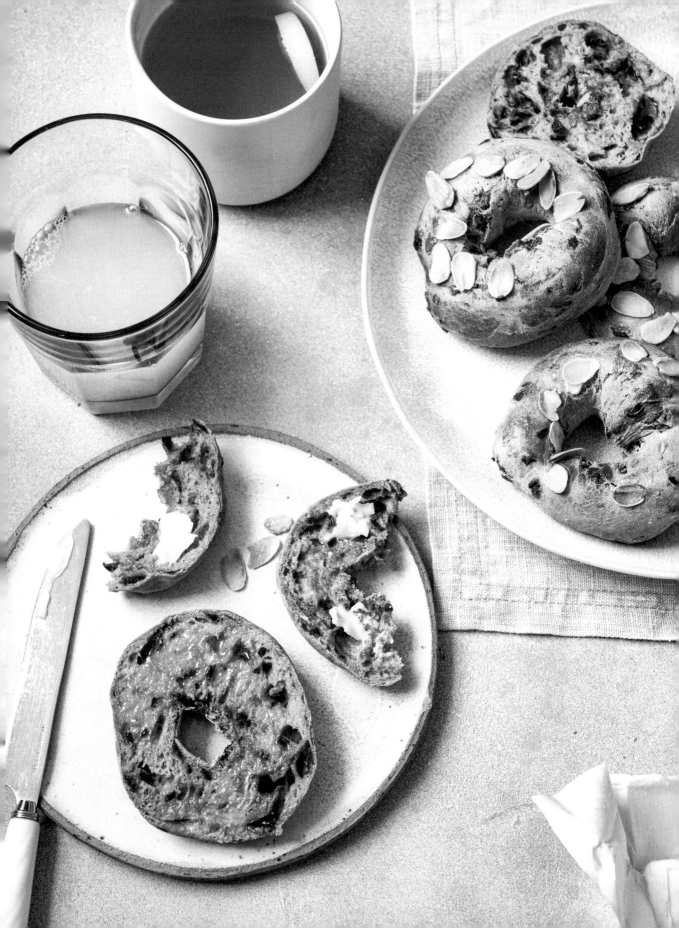

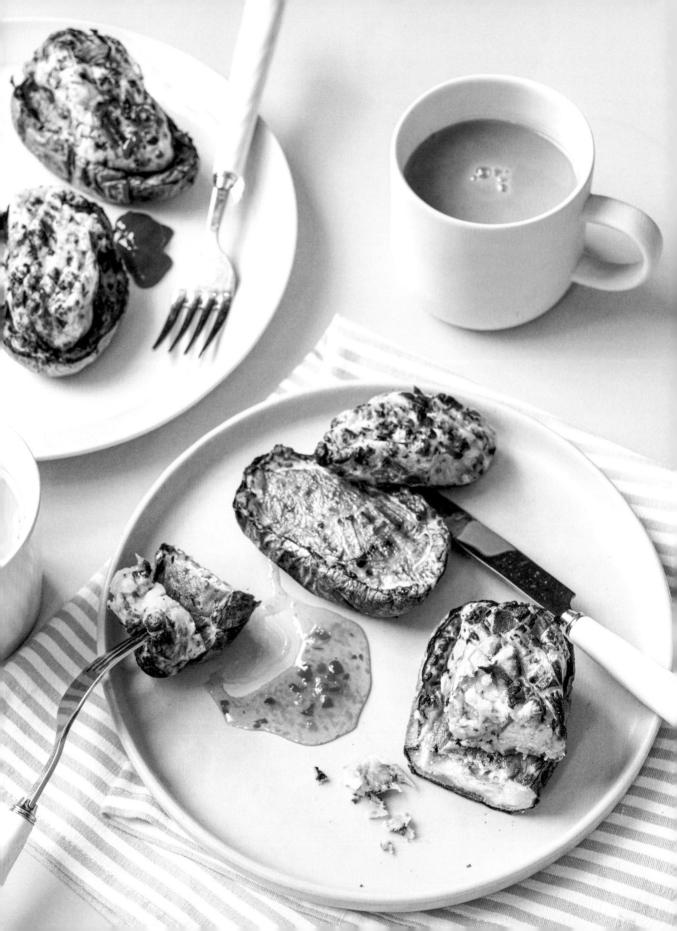

TOP HAT CRISPY POTATO SKINS

SERVES 2
PREP TIME 10 minutes
COOK TIME 50–60 minutes

2 large baking potatoes (about 250g / 9oz each)
spray oil
4 smoked bacon medallions
1 red onion, finely chopped
30g (1oz) Cheddar cheese, grated
2 eggs
salt and pepper

Crispy potato skins with a cheesy bacon-and-onion 'hat' make a savoury and satisfying breakfast or brunch. Serve with your favourite sauce: I like brown sauce with these!

1. Preheat 1 air fryer drawer to 200°C (400°F). Prick the potatoes a few times with a sharp knife, pop them in the drawer, spray with a little oil and season with salt to help them crisp up as they cook. Cook for 40–50 minutes, turning them halfway. Check that they are cooked all the way through by inserting the tip of a sharp knife into the thickest part; the inside should be tender and offer no resistance. Use silicone tongs to transfer the potatoes to a chopping board and a sharp knife to cut them in half lengthways. Leave them flesh-side up to cool a little.

2. Carefully remove the crisper plate from 1 drawer of the air fryer then preheat it to 190°C (375°F). Place the bacon medallions and red onion in the drawer and spray the onion with oil. Cook for 5 minutes. Remove the bacon and roughly chop it.

3. Scoop the middle out of each potato, leaving a little potato 'shell' inside each one. Place the scooped-out flesh into a bowl and mash it with a fork, then mash in half the cheese, onion and bacon, plus a pinch of pepper. Use your hands to shape the potato mixture into 4 ovals roughly the same size as the potato skins, pressing them firmly so they won't crumble apart. Now use a sharp knife to gently score a criss-cross pattern across the top of each oval, to help them crisp up nicely on top.

4. Crack the eggs into another bowl, lightly beat them and add the remaining cheese, onion and bacon and another pinch of pepper. Mix thoroughly. Spoon the egg mixture into the potato skins, dividing it equally between them.

5. Preheat both air fryer drawers, with the crisper plates in, to 200°C (400°F), then carefully add the potato skins (being careful not to spill the egg), and the potato ovals, ensuring a little space between each. Spray the potato ovals with oil. Cook for 8–10 minutes, until the egg is cooked through and there is a lovely golden-brown colour on the potato ovals. Use silicone tongs to gently remove the potato skins and place 2 on each plate. Use a spatula to carefully remove the potato ovals. Top each potato skin with an oval, like a little top hat.

PER SERVING

CALORIES	FAT	SAT FAT	CARBS	SUGARS	FIBRE	PROTEIN	SALT
472	14G	5.4G	51G	6.6G	5.7G	32G	3.2G

SWEET CHILLI MUSHROOMS & POACHED EGG ON TOAST

SERVES 2
PREP TIME 5 minutes
COOK TIME 16 minutes

250g (9oz) chestnut mushrooms, sliced

spray oil

2 eggs

1 tablespoon sweet chilli sauce

4 small (or 2 large) slices of wholemeal seeded bread

butter, for the toast (optional)

salt and pepper

chopped parsley leaves, to serve

Did you know that you can make perfectly poached eggs in the air fryer? You may need to experiment with your own air fryer to find its perfect cooking time for poaching them. It can depend on the size and temperature of the egg, your bakeware and the model of the air fryer. Once you have 'cracked' it, you will have perfect poached eggs every time!

This is a stress-free way to cook a filling breakfast and – importantly – that combination of sweet chilli and mushrooms is just so yummy!

1 Remove the crisper plate from 1 air fryer drawer and preheat that drawer to 190°C (375°F), then preheat the other drawer to 200°C (400°F) with the crisper plate in.

2 Put the sliced mushrooms in the 190°C (375°F) drawer and spray with oil, tossing a couple of times to coat them. Cook for 10 minutes, giving them a shake a few times during cooking.

3 Meanwhile, spray 2 ramekins (or reusable silicone baking cups) with a little oil and half fill each with boiling water. Crack an egg into each ramekin, place into the 200°C (400°F) drawer and cook for 6 minutes.

4 When the mushrooms have 1 minute remaining, add the sweet chilli sauce to them, stir well and air fry for the final minute.

5 Toast the bread, spread lightly with butter, if using, and place on 2 plates. Divide the mushrooms between the plates on top of the toast.

6 Check the poached eggs, and, if cooked to your liking, leave them to sit with the drawer open for 1 minute. Carefully lift out the ramekins (use a tea towel or oven gloves as they will be very hot). Drain the water and use a dessert spoon to carefully lift out the eggs and place on top of the mushrooms. If they have become stuck to the sides of the ramekin, carefully go around the edges with a knife to loosen them.

7 Season with salt and pepper, then sprinkle with parsley to serve.

PER SERVING

CALORIES	FAT	SAT FAT	CARBS	SUGARS	FIBRE	PROTEIN	SALT
237	9.8G	2G	19G	8G	6.5G	15G	0.64G

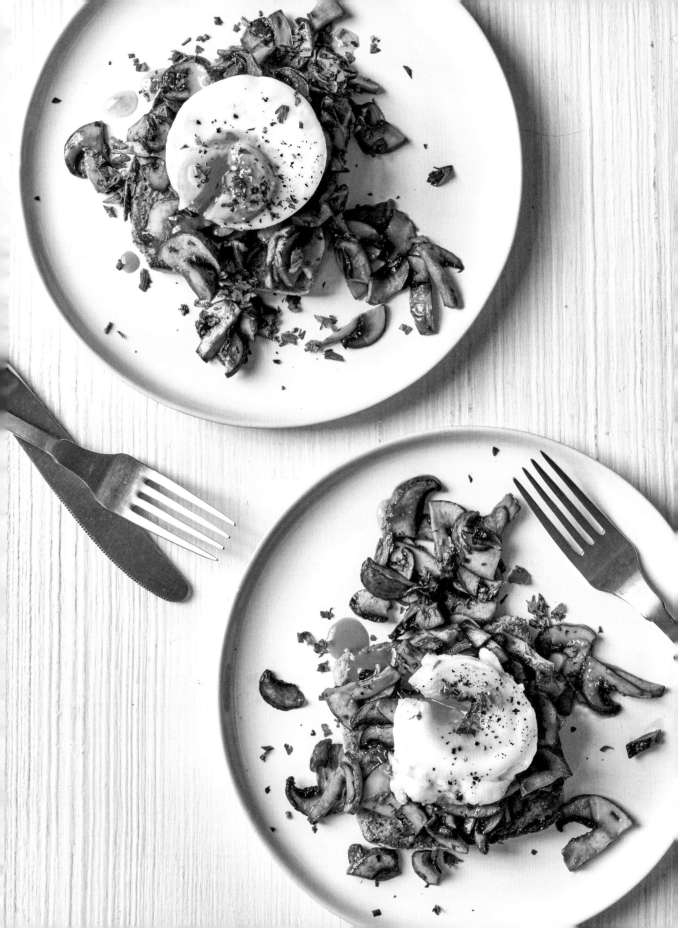

HONEY-ROAST HAM

PREP-AHEAD SEASONED
CHICKEN

TUNA & PESTO MELT

MINI HAM & MUSHROOM
QUICHES

MEDITERRANEAN-STYLE
LAMB KEBABS

SWEET 'N' SMOKY COD WITH
LEMONY WHITE BEANS

BALSAMIC-GARLIC GLAZED
SALMON

PORK & CRISPY UDON
NOODLE BALLS

PATATAS BRAVAS

RED PEPPER & CHICKPEA
PATTIES WITH LEMON
WHIPPED FETA

Lighter bites & lunches

2

HONEY-ROAST HAM

SERVES 8 (depending how you use the ham)
PREP TIME 5 minutes
COOK TIME 1 hour

750g (1lb 10oz) unsmoked gammon joint
2 tablespoons honey

Create a succulent honey-roast ham effortlessly in your air fryer with this simple recipe. Scored and glazed with honey, the gammon joint cooks to perfection, developing a caramelized exterior. Ideal for serving hot or cold, with egg, beans and chips, or for sandwiches or salads during the week, or simply as a tasty snack!

1 Preheat 1 air fryer drawer to 160°C (325°F).

2 Use a sharp knife to score a criss-cross pattern across the top of the gammon joint, lay it on a large piece of foil and drizzle it with 1 tablespoon of the honey. Wrap the foil over the ham, leaving a little space at the top between the ham and the foil so it doesn't stick to the honey, then place it in the air fryer drawer to cook.

3 After 45 minutes, remove the drawer, open the foil and drizzle over the remaining tablespoon of honey. Leave the foil open now, but make sure it's slightly pushed down so it doesn't reach to the top of the air fryer drawer. Put the drawer back into the air fryer and cook for another 10 minutes.

4 Increase the air fryer temperature to 200°C (400°F) and cook for a final 5 minutes to give it a lovely glaze.

5 I recommend using a digital food thermometer to check that your meat is thoroughly cooked all the way through: the internal temperature here should be at least 71°C (160°F).

6 Allow the ham to rest for 10 minutes before slicing it thinly.

PER SERVING

CALORIES	FAT	SAT FAT	CARBS	SUGARS	FIBRE	PROTEIN	SALT
168	5.8G	2.2G	4.4G	3.9G	0.6G	24G	2.6G

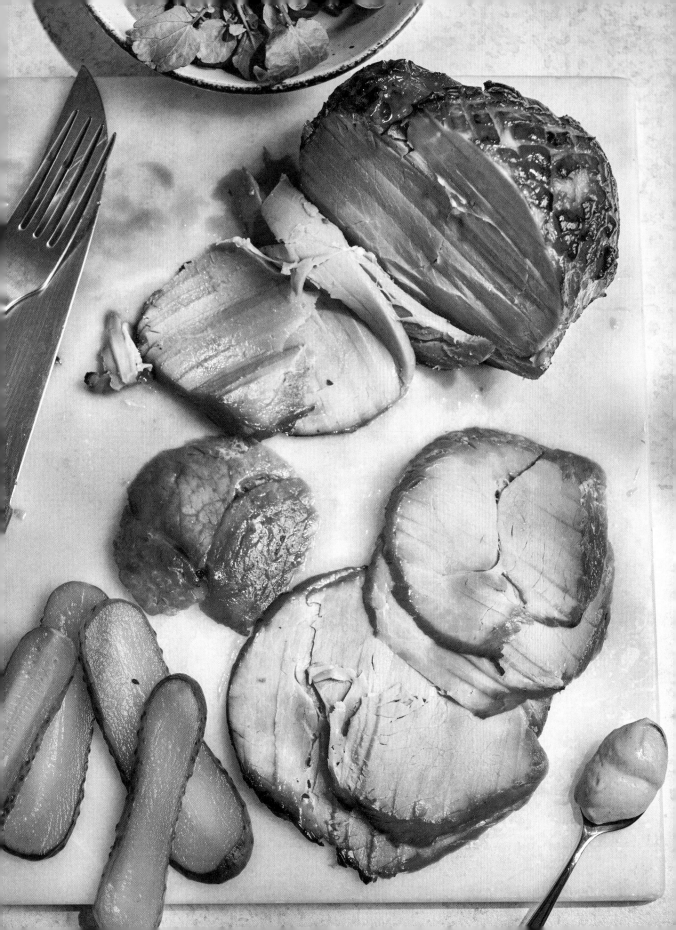

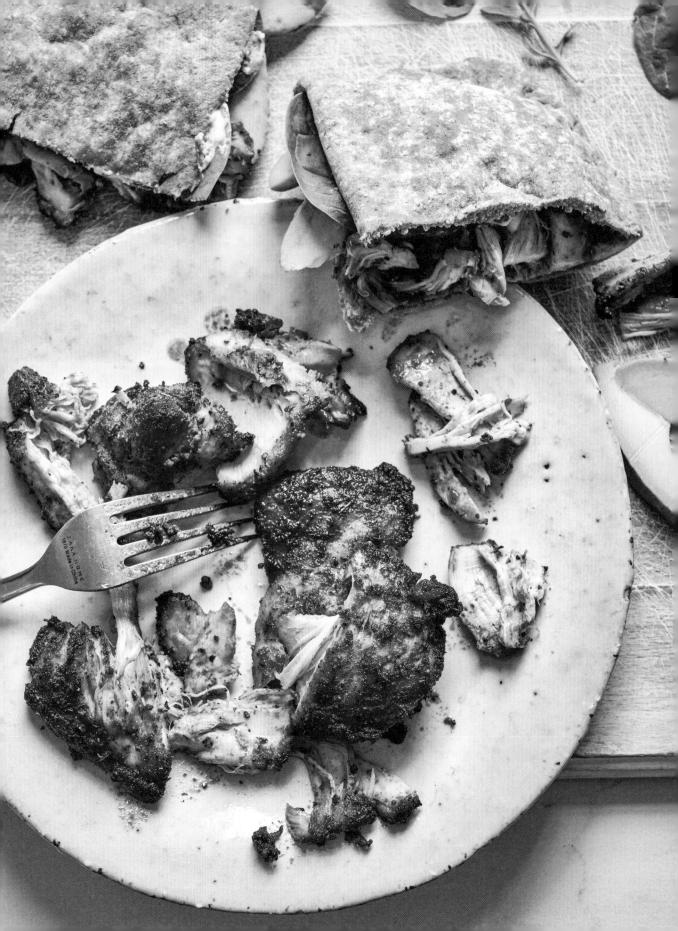

PREP-AHEAD SEASONED CHICKEN

SERVES 4
PREP TIME 10 minutes
COOK TIME 12–14 minutes

8 skinless chicken thigh fillets, excess fat trimmed away

2 tablespoons smoked paprika

1 tablespoon dried basil

1 tablespoon garlic granules

1 tablespoon onion granules or powder

1 teaspoon coarsely ground salt

1 teaspoon cracked black peppercorns

2 teaspoons olive oil

Chicken pittas are one of our go-to lunches at home and I like to have the chicken cooked and ready to go at the beginning of the week so I can quickly assemble them when needed. I buy wholemeal pitta pockets because they are nice and easy to stuff. You can fill them with whatever salad bits and pieces you have, but my favourite combination is wholemeal pitta, the inside spread with crispy chilli (I buy this online), then stuffed with thinly sliced avocado and sliced chicken.

1   Preheat both air fryer drawers to 190°C (375°F).

2   Put the chicken in a large bowl and sprinkle over all the powdered and dried seasonings. Mix everything together until the chicken thighs are coated, then drizzle over the oil and stir again to coat the chicken.

3   Lay the chicken thighs in the drawers, leaving a little space between each. Cook for 14 minutes, turning the chicken halfway to ensure that both sides are crisped. Check that the chicken is completely cooked through (the internal temperature should be at least 75°C / 167°F). You can now use the chicken as you like, warm or cold.

PER SERVING

CALORIES	FAT	SAT FAT	CARBS	SUGARS	FIBRE	PROTEIN	SALT
308	16G	4.2G	4.7G	2.2G	2G	36G	1.6G

TUNA & PESTO MELT

SERVES 4 (or 2 hungry people!)
PREP TIME 8 minutes
COOK TIME 8 minutes

2 teaspoons pesto

4 wholemeal sandwich thins
(or see recipe introduction)

145g (5oz) can of tuna in spring
water, drained

1 tablespoon reduced-fat cream
cheese

60g (2¼oz) Cheddar cheese,
grated

salt and pepper

A tuna melt is one of my favourite lunchtime choices, and the air fryer is perfect for getting the bread crispy on the outside and the cheese melty in the middle. I like these made with sandwich thins because that all-over crust gives a great crunch, but you can use whatever bread you fancy.

1   Preheat both air fryer drawers to 180°C (350°F).

2   Spread ½ teaspoon of pesto over the bottom half of each sandwich thin.

3   In a bowl, combine the tuna, cream cheese, Cheddar and salt and pepper and use a fork to thoroughly mix it. The cream cheese should help it bind together and make it easy to spread the filling over the sandwich thins without it falling out everywhere. Divide the mixture equally between the 4 sandwich thins, spreading it over the top of the pesto.

4   Add the top half of the sandwich thins and press down to stick the sandwiches together as much as possible without squashing the filling out of the edges. Place 2 tuna melts in each air fryer drawer and cook for 8 minutes. By this time the cheese should be fully melted.

5   Slice each tuna melt in half diagonally and serve. If you do slice it and find that the cheese hasn't fully melted in the middle, you can pop it back in the air fryer to cook for a couple more minutes, as being cut in half will make sure the middle cooks.

PER SERVING

CALORIES	FAT	SAT FAT	CARBS	SUGARS	FIBRE	PROTEIN	SALT
203	8.4G	4.2G	15G	1.8G	1.6G	16G	0.87G

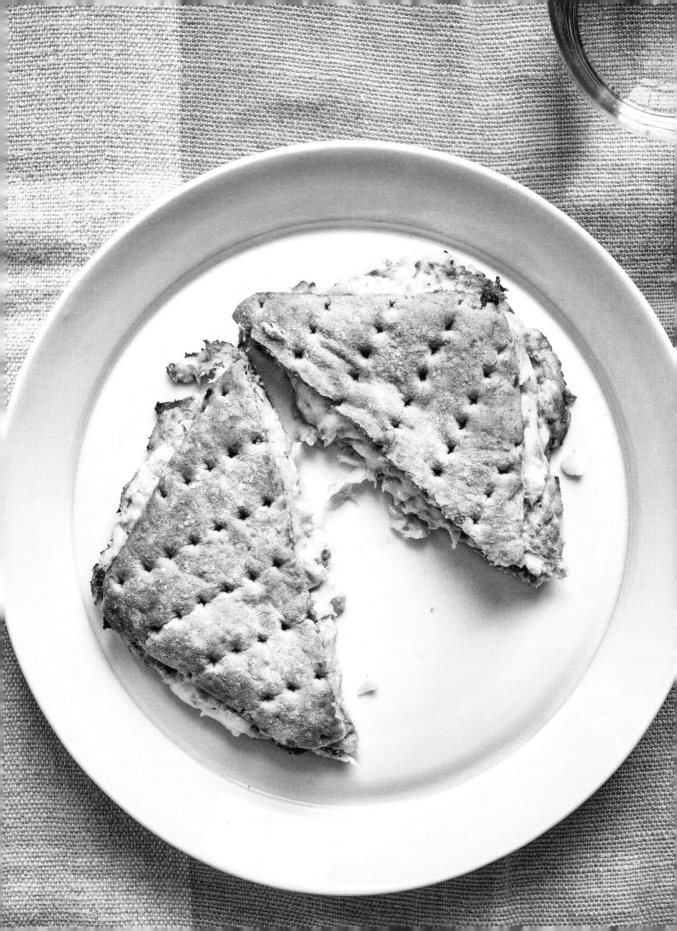

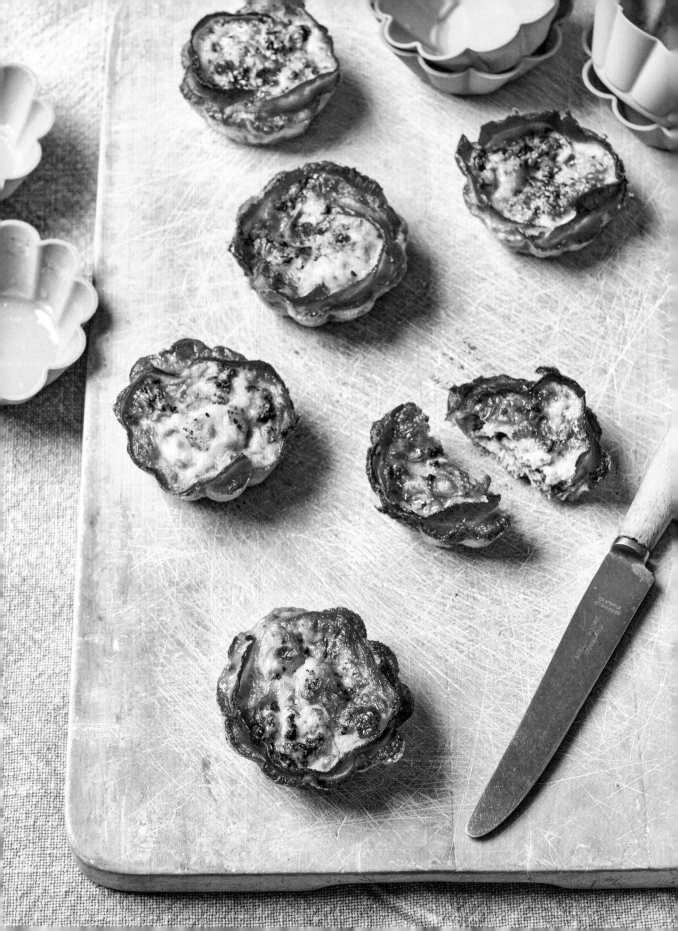

MINI HAM & MUSHROOM QUICHES

MAKES 6
PREP TIME 10 minutes
COOK TIME 15 minutes

6 slices of wafer-thin ham

2 eggs

1 tablespoon fat-free cottage cheese

pinch of black pepper

40g (1½oz) Cheddar cheese, grated

2 chestnut mushrooms, finely chopped

Use silicone cupcake moulds to make these tasty little quiches, which are perfect for lunches, snacks and picnics.

1 Preheat your air fryer to 180°C (350°F).

2 Set out 6 silicone cupcake cases. Cut each slice of ham into 4 pieces and layer them to form a lining inside the cases and to create a ham 'crust' for the quiches.

3 In a bowl, beat together the eggs and cottage cheese with a pinch of pepper, then stir in the Cheddar.

4 Divide the chopped mushrooms between the ham crusts, then spoon in the egg and cheese mix, dividing it equally between the cases and making sure it gets down into any gaps between the pieces of mushroom.

5 Place carefully into the air fryer and cook for 10–15 minutes (check them after 10 minutes). These are delicious hot or cold.

PER QUICHE

CALORIES	FAT	SAT FAT	CARBS	SUGARS	FIBRE	PROTEIN	SALT
68	4.4G	2G	0.6G	0.5G	0	6.6G	0.39G

MEDITERRANEAN-STYLE LAMB KEBABS

SERVES 2
PREP TIME 15 minutes
COOK TIME 17 minutes

---

1 red onion, cut into wedges

1 courgette, finely chopped

1 red pepper, deseeded and finely chopped

4 pickled chillies, finely chopped

2 teaspoons olive oil

2 lean lamb leg steaks, total weight 300g (10½oz) cut into strips, larger bits of fat trimmed away

2 teaspoons sweet paprika

1 teaspoon dried oregano

½ teaspoon sumac

¼ teaspoon ground turmeric

½ teaspoon coarsely ground salt

2 tablespoons tomato purée

juice of 1 lemon

3 garlic cloves, crushed

2 large wholemeal tortillas or pittas (I like the easy-stuff soft wholemeal pittas)

FOR THE MINT YOGURT SAUCE

small handful of mint leaves, finely chopped

4 tablespoons fat-free Greek yogurt

pinch of coarsely ground salt

This delicious lamb mixture is packed full of flavour for an impressively easy lunch. I serve it in wholemeal pittas, but you can use tortillas or flatbreads if you prefer, or just serve the lamb alongside rice, couscous or salad.

1 Remove the crisper plates and preheat 1 air fryer drawer to 180°C (350°F) and the other to 200°C (400°F).

2 Put the onion in the 200°C (400°F) drawer with the courgette, pepper, pickled chillies and 1 teaspoon of the olive oil. Cook for 17 minutes, stirring about every 4 minutes.

3 Mix together the lamb, spices, herbs and salt, tomato purée, lemon juice, garlic and remaining 1 teaspoon of olive oil. Place in the 180°C (350°F) drawer and cook for 12 minutes, stirring every 4 minutes.

4 Meanwhile, make the sauce by mixing the chopped mint and salt into the yogurt in a small bowl. Warm the tortillas or toast the pitta breads.

5 Once everything is cooked, mix the lamb mixture with the vegetables.

6 Spread the mint yogurt on each tortilla or inside each pitta and stuff with the lamb kebab filling.

PER SERVING

CALORIES	FAT	SAT FAT	CARBS	SUGARS	FIBRE	PROTEIN	SALT
332	5.6G	0.9G	47G	16G	10G	17	2.9G

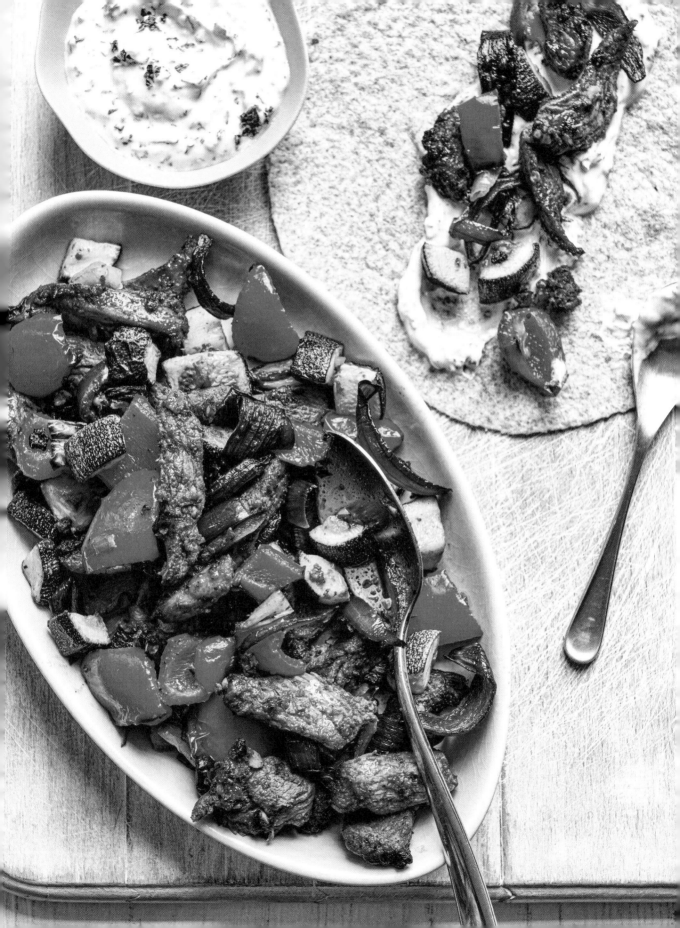

SWEET 'N' SMOKY COD WITH LEMONY WHITE BEANS

SERVES 4
PREP TIME 30 minutes
(including marinating time)
COOK TIME 10 minutes

Tender cod fillets coated with a vibrant sweet and smoky marinade and served with zesty lemon and garlic white beans makes a delicious, summery meal. Serve this with seasonal greens; asparagus, ribbons of courgette or green beans work well. For a special touch, crisp and salty samphire makes a perfect accompaniment.

2 garlic cloves, crushed

2 tablespoons red wine vinegar

2 teaspoons smoked paprika

1 teaspoon tomato purée

1 teaspoon honey

1 teaspoon olive oil

4 x 400–500g (14oz–1lb 2oz) cod, or similar firm white fish fillets

salt and pepper

FOR THE LEMONY BEANS

2 garlic cloves, crushed

juice and finely grated zest of 1 lemon

400g (14oz) can of cannellini beans, drained and rinsed

400g (14oz) can of butter beans, drained and rinsed

1 teaspoon olive oil

100ml (3½fl oz) hot chicken stock

small handful of finely chopped parsley leaves, plus more to serve

½ teaspoon coarsely ground salt

1   In a bowl, mix the garlic, vinegar, smoked paprika, tomato purée, honey and olive oil, then season with salt and pepper. Pat the cod fillets dry with kitchen paper and place them in the marinade, spooning some over the top to make sure they are completely coated. Cover the bowl and leave to marinate for at least 15 minutes, or up to 1 hour.

2   Meanwhile, for the beans, put the garlic into a small bowl with the lemon juice (make sure you have zested the lemon first). Leave this for the same amount of time as the fish, to mellow the potency of the garlic.

3   Preheat 1 air fryer drawer to 200°C (400°F) with the crisper plate in, and the other drawer to 180°C (350°F) with the crisper plate removed.

4   Mix the beans, olive oil, hot stock and the garlic mixture and spoon into the 180°C (350°F) drawer. Air fry for 10 minutes, stirring every few minutes.

5   Place the fish fillets in the 200°C (400°F) drawer, ensuring there is space between each. You should be able to fit in all 4 fillets, but, if necessary, cook in batches. Air fry for 8–10 minutes, depending on thickness. To check if the fish is cooked, either use a thermometer to ensure the thickest part of the fillet has reached at least 63°C (145°F), or cut into a fillet to ensure it is cooked through: it should look opaque and flake apart in the middle.

6   Once the beans are cooked, stir through the lemon zest and parsley, then season with the salt and a good grinding of pepper. Serve the fish fillets over the beans, with a scattering of extra parsley.

PER PORTION

CALORIES	FAT	SAT FAT	CARBS	SUGARS	FIBRE	PROTEIN	SALT
244	3.5G	0.5G	21G	1.8G	9.6G	27G	1.1G

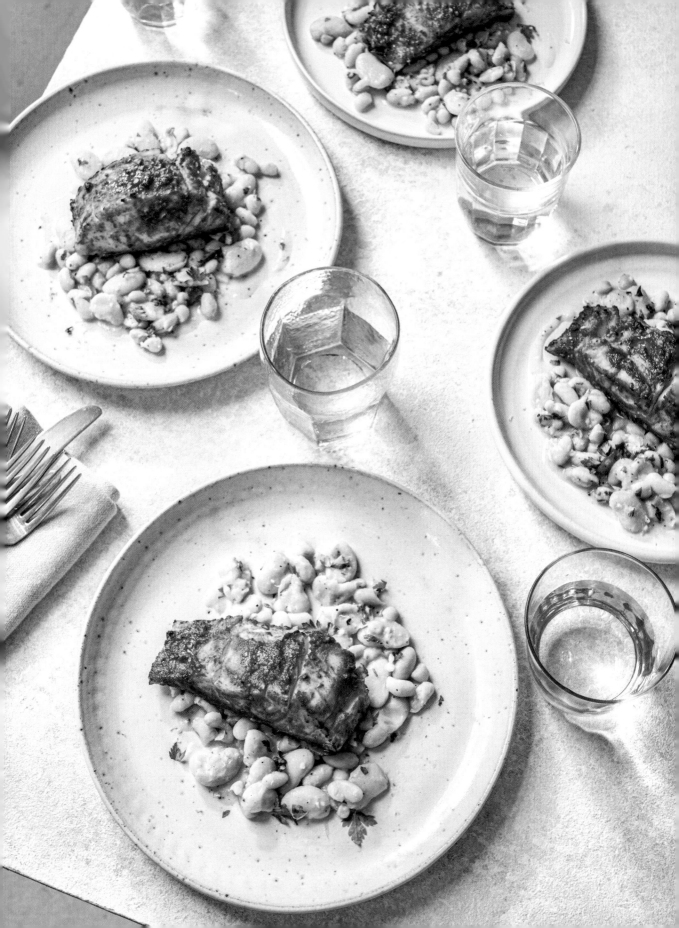

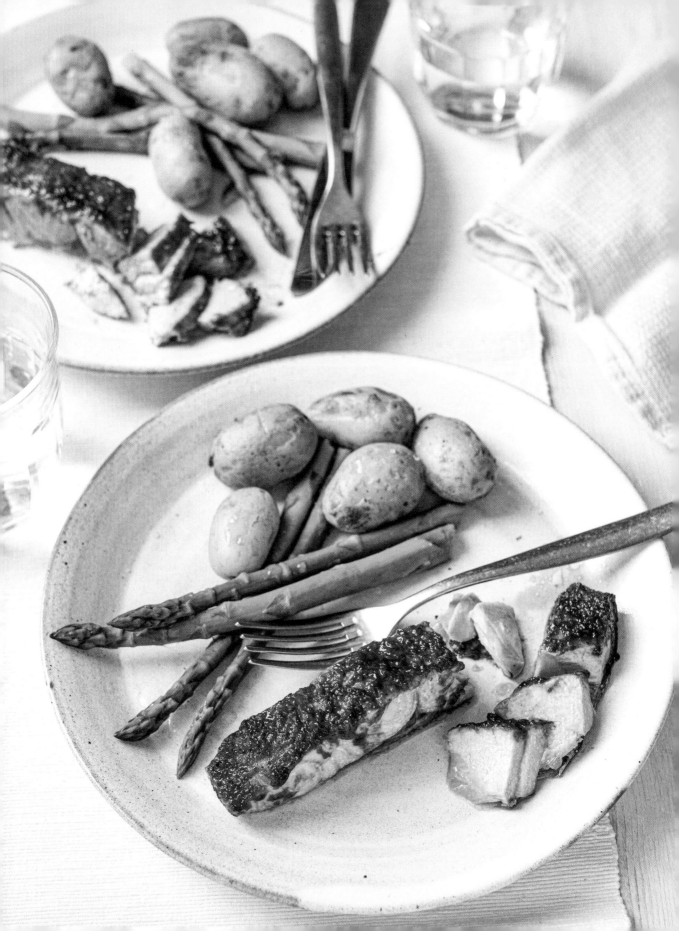

BALSAMIC-GARLIC GLAZED SALMON

SERVES 4
PREP TIME 5 minutes
COOK TIME 10 minutes

1 tablespoon balsamic vinegar

1 tablespoon honey

1 tablespoon Dijon mustard

2 garlic cloves, crushed

¼ teaspoon coarsely ground salt

¼ teaspoon cracked black peppercorns

4 salmon fillets

This flavour-packed balsamic glaze perfectly complements the tender salmon fillets. I serve these with in-season new potatoes and asparagus, or a simple salad.

1   In a small bowl, mix the balsamic vinegar, honey, mustard, garlic, salt and pepper. Lay the salmon fillets on a plate and use a teaspoon to spread the glaze over the top.

2   Preheat both air fryer drawers to 180°C (350°F).

3   Lay 2 fish fillets in each drawer and spoon any remaining glaze over the top. Air fry for 8–10 minutes (thicker fillets need 10 minutes). When they are cooked, the exterior should be lovely and caramelized and the salmon will be an opaque pink colour and easily flake into distinct layers if you insert a fork into the thickest part.

PER SERVING

CALORIES	FAT	SAT FAT	CARBS	SUGARS	FIBRE	PROTEIN	SALT
308	20G	3.6G	4.3G	4G	0.5G	27G	0.71G

PORK & CRISPY UDON NOODLE BALLS

SERVES 4
PREP TIME 5 minutes
COOK TIME 15 minutes

300g (10½oz) ready-cooked udon noodles, cut into 2–3cm (1 inch) lengths

300g (10½oz) 5 per cent fat minced pork

6 spring onions, finely chopped

2 garlic cloves, crushed

handful of finely chopped coriander

2 tablespoons oyster sauce

1 tablespoon fish sauce

juice and finely grated zest of 1 lime

spray oil

FOR THE DIPPING SAUCE

3 tablespoons sweet chilli sauce

2 tablespoons light soy sauce

1 tablespoon rice vinegar

Everyone in my family loves these flavour-bombs. We serve them with Fried edamame (see page 152), or, to make them more of a meal, with a slaw-style salad with crunchy veg – such as shredded red cabbage and carrot dressed with lime juice – or simply some crisp Little Gem lettuce leaves.

1 In a large bowl, mix the noodles, pork, spring onions, garlic, coriander, oyster sauce, fish sauce and lime zest. Mix thoroughly and then use your hands to combine the mixture even further. Roll the mixture into equal balls, each around 4cm, pressing firmly as you make them to keep them together, then place on a plate. The quantities here should make 16 balls.

2 Preheat both air fryer drawers to 180°C (350°F).

3 Divide the noodle balls between the drawers, transferring them carefully so as not to break them apart. Spray them with oil, then cook for 15 minutes. I don't turn these halfway through, to avoid breaking them. After 15 minutes, they should be cooked through, with some lovely crispy bits of noodle on the outside.

4 Meanwhile, make the dipping sauce by stirring all the ingredients in a small bowl with the lime juice.

5 Serve the noodle balls with the dipping sauce on the side.

PER SERVING

CALORIES	FAT	SAT FAT	CARBS	SUGARS	FIBRE	PROTEIN	SALT
242	3.8G	0.7G	24G	5G	3G	25G	3.4G

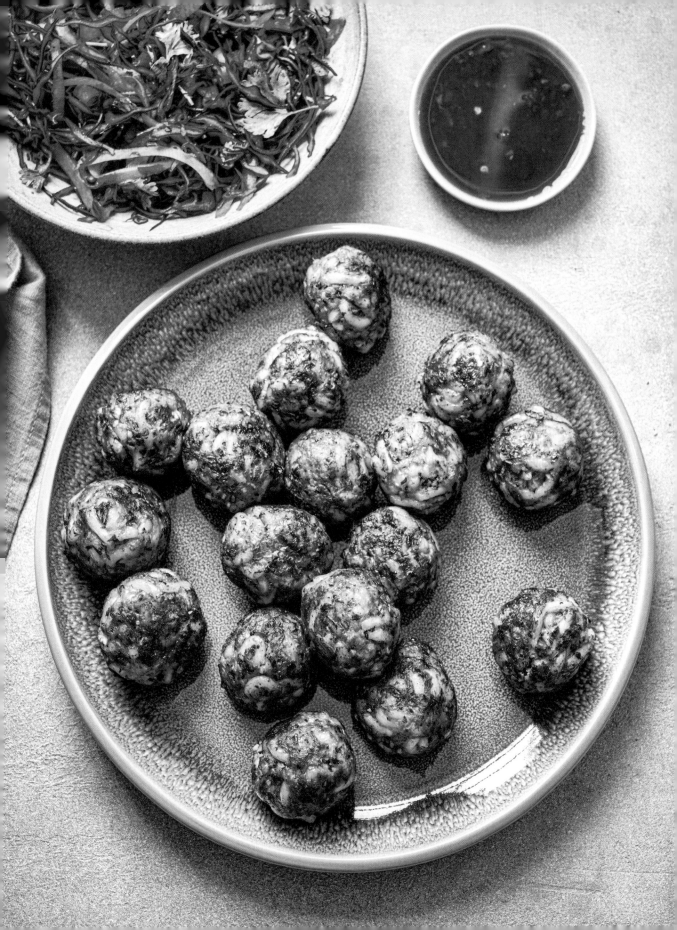

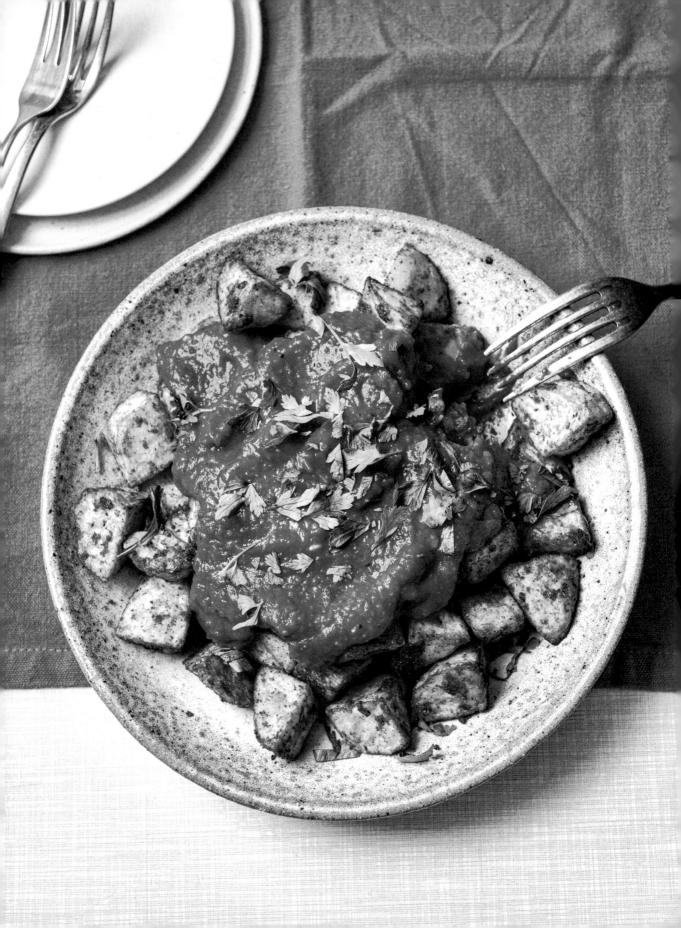

PATATAS BRAVAS

SERVES 4
PREP TIME 15 minutes
COOK TIME 30 minutes

800g (1lb 12oz) Maris Piper or other white floury potatoes, peeled and cut into 2–3cm (1 inch) cubes
1 tablespoon olive oil
1 tablespoon smoked paprika
1 tablespoon garlic granules
salt and pepper

FOR THE SAUCE
1 red onion, finely chopped
2 garlic cloves, finely chopped
½ red chilli, deseeded and finely chopped
1 teaspoon olive oil
250ml (9fl oz) tomato passata
1 tablespoon white wine vinegar
½ teaspoon smoked paprika
¼ teaspoon dried oregano
finely chopped parsley, to serve

My take on the famous Spanish tapas dish utilizes the air fryer for those hot, crispy potatoes smothered in a deliciously piquant tomato sauce.

1   Soak the potato cubes in cold water for 10 minutes, then drain and pat dry with kitchen paper. Put them in a mixing bowl with the olive oil, smoked paprika, garlic granules, salt and pepper and stir until coated.

2   Preheat both air fryer drawers to 180°C (350°F).

3   Divide the potatoes evenly between the 2 drawers and cook for 20 minutes, shaking every 5 minutes. Transfer all the potatoes to the mixing bowl.

4   Carefully remove the crisper plate from one of the drawers and add the onion, chopped garlic, chilli and olive oil; stir then cook for 5 minutes. Add the passata, vinegar, smoked paprika and oregano, season with salt and pepper, stir and cook for 15 minutes, stirring every 5 minutes.

5   When there are 10 minutes remaining on the sauce, preheat the empty air fryer drawer containing the crisper plate to 200°C (400°F). Add the potatoes and cook for 10 minutes, shaking every now and again. You want to ensure the potatoes are hot and crispy, but check to ensure they aren't burning.

6   Once the sauce is ready, transfer it to a mini food processor and blend until smooth.

7   Serve the potatoes with the sauce poured over and scattered with parsley.

PER SERVING

CALORIES	FAT	SAT FAT	CARBS	SUGARS	FIBRE	PROTEIN	SALT
252	4.8G	0.6G	42G	7.7G	4.5G	6.4G	0.16G

RED PEPPER & CHICKPEA PATTIES WITH LEMON WHIPPED FETA

SERVES 4
PREP TIME 20 minutes
COOK TIME 14 minutes

These tasty little patties, like falafels, are elevated to the next level with light and creamy whipped feta spiked with zesty lemon and topped with fresh herbs. They make a great snack, or are ideal to serve with salad or grains.

400g (14oz) can of chickpeas, drained and rinsed
1 red pepper, deseeded and roughly chopped
1 onion, finely chopped
1 carrot, roughly chopped
1 garlic clove, cut into a few pieces
1 teaspoon ground cumin
1 teaspoon smoked paprika
½ teaspoon chilli flakes
1 egg, lightly beaten
2 tablespoons chia seeds
spray oil
salt and pepper

FOR THE WHIPPED FETA
200g (7oz) feta cheese
60g (2¼oz) fat-free Greek yogurt
finely grated zest of 1 lemon and juice of ½
1 teaspoon olive oil
small handful of mixed herbs, such as mint, parsley and thyme leaves, finely chopped
cracked black peppercorns

1 Put the chickpeas in a food processor with the red pepper, onion, carrot, garlic, cumin, smoked paprika, chilli flakes and salt and pepper, then pulse-blend to chop everything into a slightly chunky mixture, without completely puréeing. Mix through the egg and chia seeds.

2 Preheat both air fryer drawers to 200°C (400°F).

3 Form the chickpea mixture into 16 balls, each about 1 tablespoon.

4 Carefully line the hot drawers with nonstick baking paper, spray with a little oil, and place the balls directly on the baking paper in the drawers. Use a fork to gently press each into a slightly flattened circle. Spray with oil, then cook for 14 minutes.

5 Meanwhile, to make the whipped feta, place the feta, yogurt, most of the lemon zest (reserve a little to serve), the lemon juice and olive oil in a mini food processor or blender and whizz until smooth with a 'whipped' consistency, a bit like whipped cream, only thicker. Don't be tempted to blend it further as this can make it too runny. Scrape into a small bowl and stir in the cracked black peppercorns, the remaining lemon zest and most of the herbs (saving some for garnish).

6 Serve the chickpea patties with the whipped feta, scattered with the remaining herbs.

PER SERVING

CALORIES	FAT	SAT FAT	CARBS	SUGARS	FIBRE	PROTEIN	SALT
292	16G	7.7G	17G	5.8G	7.6G	17G	1.4G

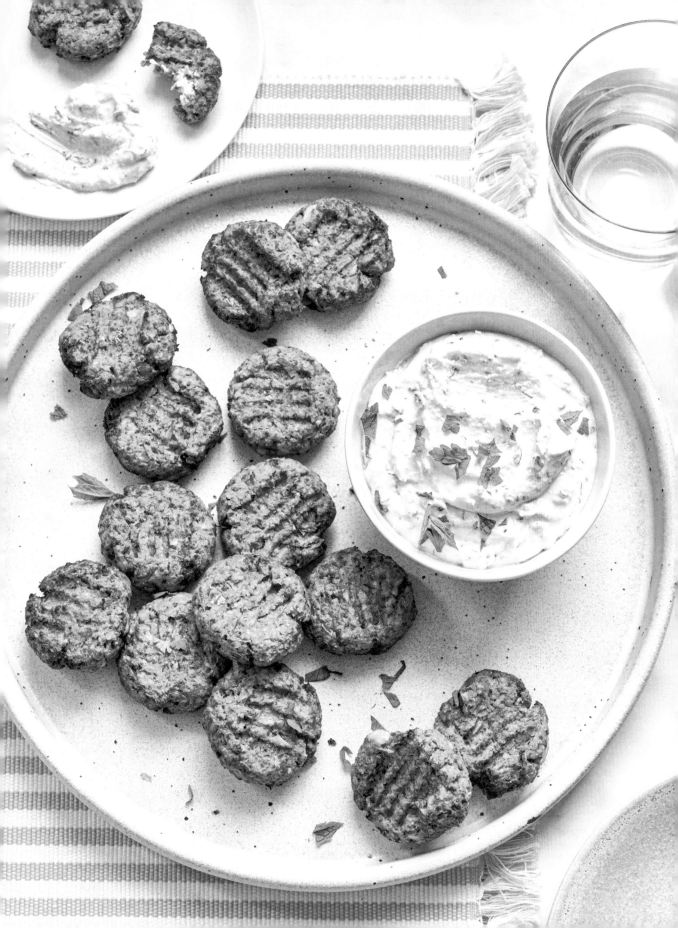

SPICED CHICKPEA &
HALLOUMI SALAD

EASY MUSHROOM SOUP

ROASTED RED PEPPER &
COCONUT SOUP

PUMPKIN-SPICE BUTTERNUT
SQUASH & PECAN SALAD

CHEESEBURGER SALAD WITH
SPECIAL SAUCE

SPECIAL SAUSAGES &
BUTTERNUT SQUASH SALAD

ROASTED CAULIFLOWER &
PISTACHIO PESTO GRAIN
SALAD

3

Soup
& salads

SPICED CHICKPEA & HALLOUMI SALAD

SERVES 4
PREP TIME 15 minutes
COOK TIME 28 minutes

2 x 400g (14oz) cans of chickpeas, drained and rinsed

1 teaspoon olive oil

1 teaspoon garam masala

1 teaspoon smoked paprika

1 teaspoon coarsely sea salt

¼ teaspoon ground cinnamon

¼ teaspoon ground turmeric

¼ teaspoon cracked black peppercorns

FOR THE SALAD

2 onions, finely sliced into half-moons

2 red, yellow or orange peppers, deseeded and finely sliced

spray oil

50g (1¾oz) sundried tomatoes, drained and finely chopped

4 garlic cloves, crushed

225g (8oz) halloumi cheese, thickly sliced

½ red cabbage, very thinly sliced

handful of parsley stalks and leaves, finely chopped

handful of basil leaves, shredded

1 tablespoon sumac

1 tablespoon red wine vinegar

juice of 1 lemon

½ teaspoon chilli powder

½ teaspoon ground cumin

salt and pepper

A hearty salad that is filling and delicious. You can eat this warm or cold, so it's perfect for either a light dinner or an easy lunch.

1 Remove the crisper plate from 1 air fryer drawer, then preheat both drawers to 200°C (400°F).

2 Mix the chickpeas with the oil and all the spices. Put them in the air fryer drawer containing the crisper plate, then cook for 10 minutes, giving them a shake a couple of times while they are cooking.

3 Put the onions and peppers in the other drawer, spray with oil, toss to coat and cook for 18 minutes, stirring a couple of times during cooking. For the last 2 minutes of cooking time, stir in the sundried tomatoes and garlic.

4 Once the chickpeas are done, transfer them to a mixing bowl.

5 Lay the halloumi slices in a single layer in the empty air fryer drawer containing the crisper plate. Cook, again at 200°C (400°F), for 10 minutes, turning halfway through.

6 To the bowl containing the chickpeas add the cabbage, parsley, basil, sumac, vinegar, lemon juice, chilli powder and ground cumin and toss to combine. Next add the cooked peppers and onions and toss again.

7 Arrange the salad on a serving platter, top with the cooked halloumi and season with salt and pepper before serving.

PER SERVING

CALORIES	FAT	SAT FAT	CARBS	SUGARS	FIBRE	PROTEIN	SALT
371	17G	9.9G	26G	13G	12G	22G	3.6G

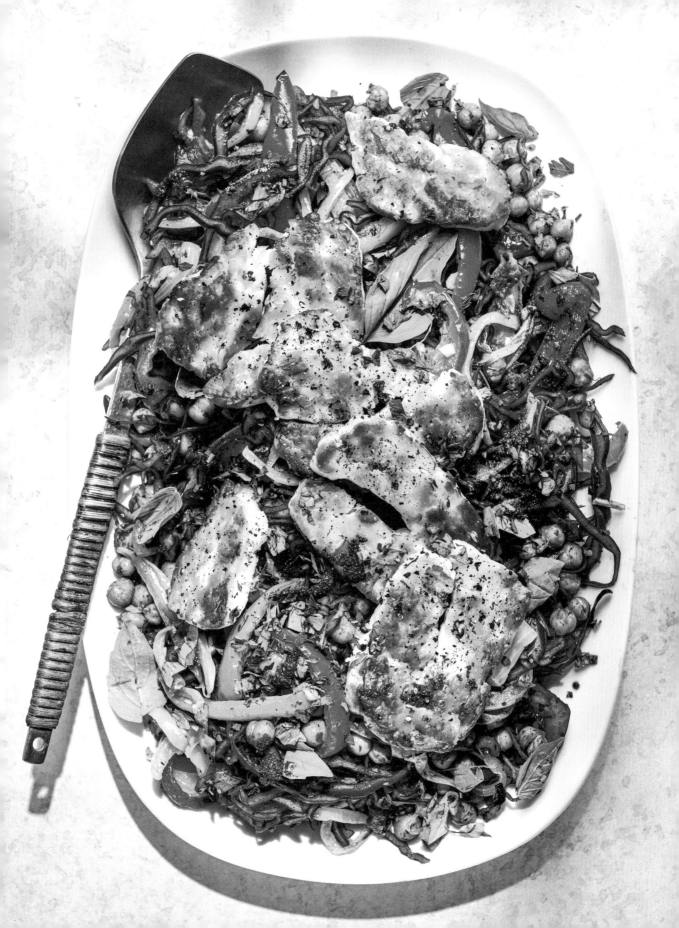

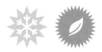

EASY MUSHROOM SOUP

SERVES 2
PREP TIME 10 minutes
COOK TIME 20 minutes

300g (10½oz) chestnut
mushrooms, finely chopped

2 garlic cloves, finely chopped

8–10 sage leaves, finely chopped,
plus more to serve

2 small onions, finely chopped

1 tablespoon olive oil

100ml (3½fl oz) semi-skimmed
milk

500ml (18fl oz) hot vegetable
stock

salt and pepper

pinch of paprika, to serve

A quick lunchtime win, which can be thrown together at a moment's
notice with a few simple ingredients.

1 Remove the crisper plate from 1 air fryer drawer, then preheat that
drawer to 180°C (350°F).

2 Put the mushrooms in the drawer, followed by the garlic and sage,
then the onions on top, and drizzle all over with the olive oil.
Cook for 15 minutes, stirring every few minutes.

3 Pour in the milk, stir thoroughly and cook for 5 more minutes.

4 Transfer the mushroom mixture to a food processor or blender, add
the hot stock and whizz it into a smooth soup. (If you have a stick
blender you can blend it directly in the drawer.) Season with salt
and pepper to taste.

5 Mushroom soup isn't always the most appetizing colour, so I usually
sprinkle servings with extra sage, a sprinkle of paprika and a grind of
black pepper to get it looking as delicious as it tastes!

PER SERVING

CALORIES	FAT	SAT FAT	CARBS	SUGARS	FIBRE	PROTEIN	SALT
159	9.3G	2.1G	9.9G	8.2G	4.5G	6.6G	0.48G

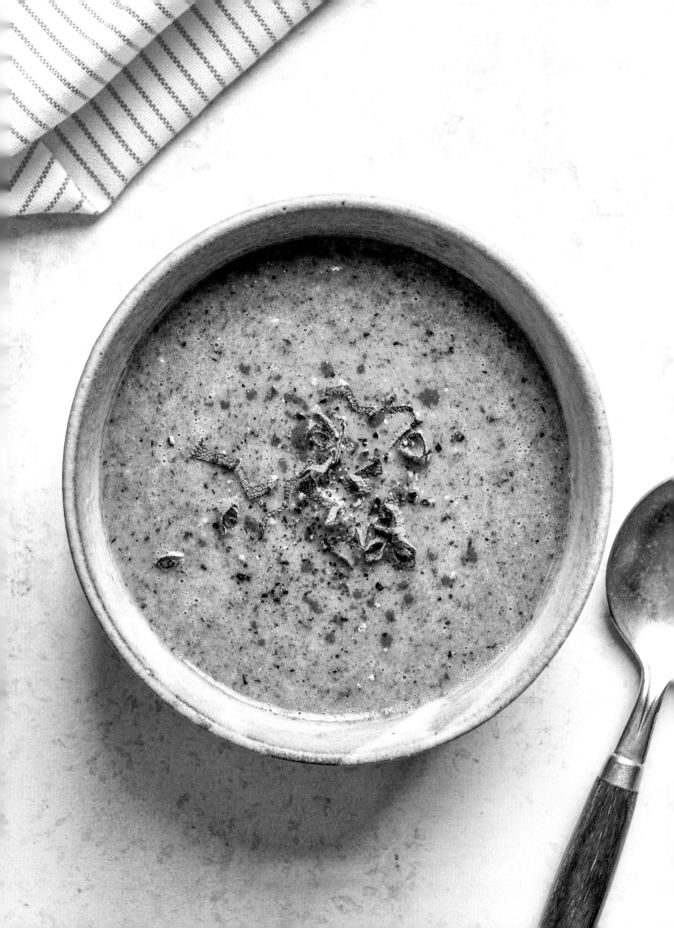

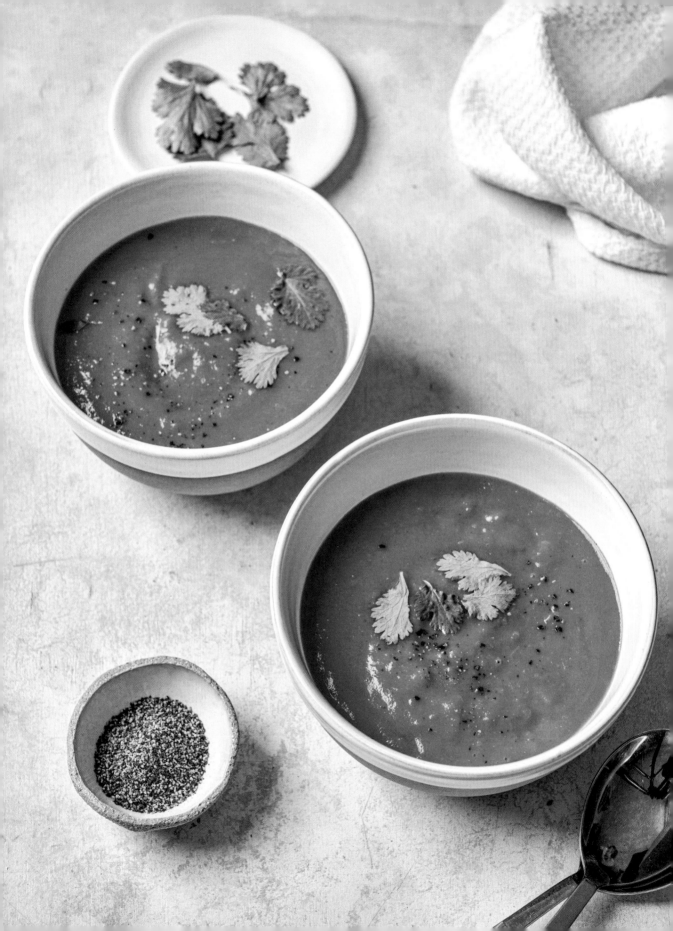

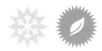

ROASTED RED PEPPER & COCONUT SOUP

SERVES 4
PREP TIME 10 minutes
COOK TIME 20 minutes

4 red peppers, deseeded and
   roughly chopped
1 large onion, sliced into wedges
spray oil
½ teaspoon ground coriander
½ teaspoon ground ginger
400g (14oz) can of chopped
   tomatoes
400g (14oz) can of reduced-fat
   coconut milk
1 tablespoon sweet chilli sauce
1 teaspoon coarsely ground salt
handful of coriander leaves
cracked black peppercorns

A rich and creamy comfort-food soup, with sweet roasted peppers and coconut milk, this makes for a luxurious lunch.

1   Remove the crisper plates and preheat both air fryer drawers to 200°C (400°F).

2   Divide the peppers and onion equally between the 2 drawers and spray with oil. Cook for 15 minutes, stirring a couple of times during the cooking time.

3   Transfer all the onion and peppers into 1 drawer, stir through the ground coriander and ginger, then add the chopped tomatoes, coconut milk, sweet chilli sauce and salt. Stir well and cook for 5 more minutes.

4   Stir again then transfer the mixture to a food processor or blender and whizz into a smooth soup. (If you have a stick blender you can blend it directly in the drawer.)

5   Divide between warmed bowls and scatter with coriander and black pepper to serve.

PER SERVING

CALORIES	FAT	SAT FAT	CARBS	SUGARS	FIBRE	PROTEIN	SALT
177	7.2G	5.6G	21G	18G	6.2G	3.6G	1.3G

PUMPKIN-SPICE BUTTERNUT SQUASH & PECAN SALAD

SERVES 4
PREP TIME 20 minutes
COOK TIME 18 minutes

1 butternut squash, chopped into 1.5cm (⅝ inch) cubes (total weight about 600g / 1lb 5oz once prepared)
1 tablespoon honey
2 teaspoons olive oil
½ teaspoon coarsely ground salt
75g (2¾oz) pecans, roughly chopped
120g (4¼oz) baby spinach leaves
80g (2¾oz) pomegranate seeds

FOR THE PUMPKIN SPICE BLEND
3 tablespoons ground cinnamon
1½ tablespoons ground ginger
2 teaspoons ground allspice
2 teaspoons ground nutmeg
½ teaspoon ground cloves

FOR THE DRESSING
juice of 1 lime
1 teaspoon olive oil
1 teaspoon honey
¼ teaspoon coarsely ground salt
½ teaspoon cracked black pepper
1 tablespoon poppy seeds

The essence of autumn cosiness: tender, sweet and spiced butternut squash cubes air fried to perfection and served with lightly toasted pecans and juicy pomegranate seeds.

The pumpkin spice mix can also be used to jazz up porridge or baked oats, or try sprinkling it on your latte or hot chocolate.

1 Put all the spices for the pumpkin spice blend in a clean jam jar and shake to combine.

2 Put the squash in a mixing bowl with 2 teaspoons of the pumpkin spice mix, plus the honey, olive oil and salt. Stir well.

3 Preheat both air fryer drawers to 200°C (400°F).

4 Divide the squash equally between the 2 drawers and shake into a single layer. Cook for 18 minutes, shaking a couple of times during cooking. For the final 2 minutes of cooking, add the chopped pecans to 1 of the drawers.

5 Tip the cooked squash and pecans onto a large platter and leave to cool for 10 minutes while you prepare the rest of the salad.

6 Make the dressing by mixing together all the ingredients in small bowl.

7 Once the air fryer drawers have cooled, carefully take out the crisper plates (they will be hot) to rescue any rogue pecan pieces and add them to the bowl. Add the spinach leaves and pomegranate seeds and toss everything together. Pour over the dressing, toss again and serve.

PER SERVING

CALORIES	FAT	SAT FAT	CARBS	SUGARS	FIBRE	PROTEIN	SALT
277	18G	1.7G	21G	15G	5G	5.1G	0.91G

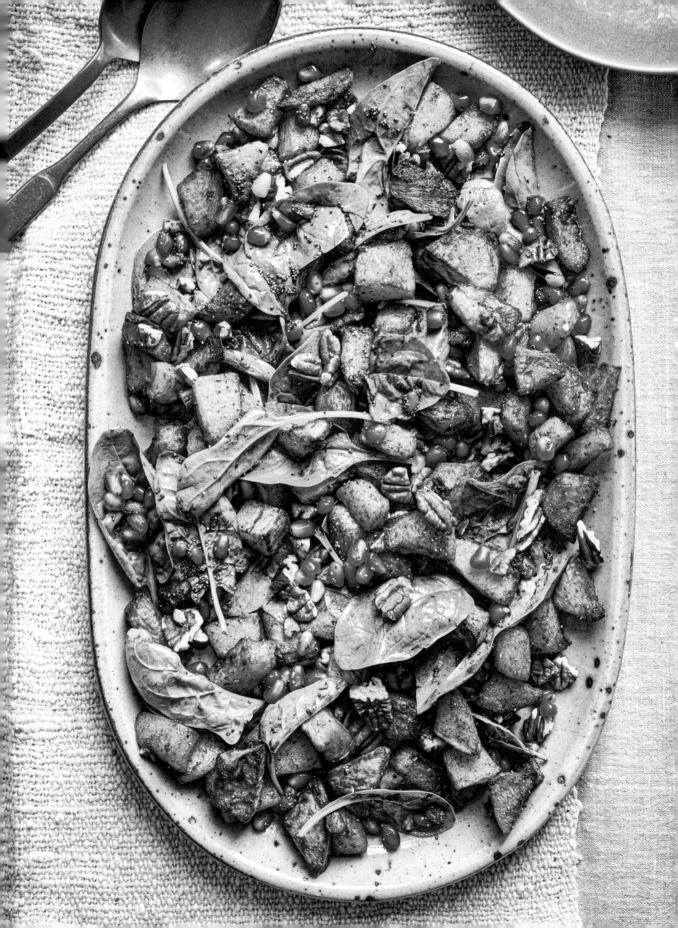

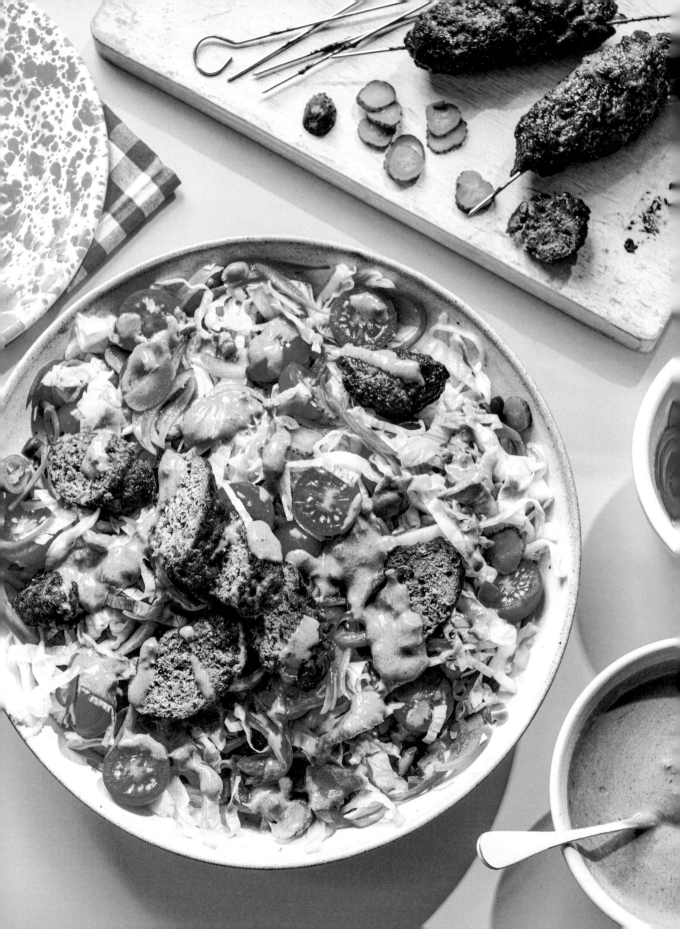

SERVES 4
PREP TIME 25 minutes
COOK TIME 16 minutes

500g (1lb 2oz) 5 per cent fat minced beef
1 tablespoon American mustard
1 tablespoon tomato ketchup
1 teaspoon onion granules
1 teaspoon garlic granules
½ teaspoon coarsely ground salt
¼ teaspoon cracked black peppercorns
1 gherkin, finely chopped
1 tablespoon Worcestershire sauce
60g (2¼oz) Cheddar cheese, grated

FOR THE SALAD

1 red onion, thinly sliced
2 tablespoons red wine vinegar
¼ teaspoon coarsely ground salt
1 Iceberg lettuce, finely shredded
400g (14oz) cherry tomatoes, halved
2 gherkins, thinly sliced
1 tablespoon pickled jalapeños, finely chopped (optional)

FOR THE SPECIAL SAUCE

100g (3½oz) fat-free Greek yogurt
juice of 1 lemon
2 tablespoons tomato purée
2 teaspoons small-chunk pickle, such as Branston
1 teaspoon honey
½ teaspoon garlic granules
¼ teaspoon paprika
¼ teaspoon coarsely ground salt
¼ teaspoon cracked black peppercorns

CHEESEBURGER SALAD WITH SPECIAL SAUCE

Here is a light twist on a classic cheeseburger that still retains its satisfying flavours in a bowl of salad. This is great on its own, but you could always serve it with homemade fries. You will need metal kebab skewers that fit in your air fryer for this recipe – I used 20cm (8 inch) skewers, but please check the dimensions of your air fryer drawers to ensure your skewers will fit.

1 Start by quick-pickling the onion for the salad. Place the thinly sliced red onion in a small bowl with the red wine vinegar and salt, then set aside to marinate.

2 Place the beef, mustard, ketchup, onion and garlic granules, salt, pepper, gherkin, Worcestershire sauce and cheese in a bowl and mix thoroughly with a fork. Break down any clumps in the beef as you go. Squeeze the meat mixture into 6 sausage shapes around 6 skewers (see recipe introduction). Try to make these similar sizes, about 100g (3½oz) each, and pack the meat as firmly as you can around each skewer.

3 Preheat both air fryer drawers to 180°C (350°F). Place 3 cheeseburger skewers in each drawer and cook for 16 minutes, carefully turning halfway through.

4 Meanwhile, toss the lettuce, tomatoes, gherkins and jalapeños together in a large serving bowl.

5 For the special sauce, mix all the ingredients in a bowl.

6 When the skewers are cooked, add the quick-pickled onion to the salad, lay the kebabs on top and drizzle with some of the sauce, serving the rest on the side so everyone can help themselves. Alternatively, you can slice up the beef kebabs and toss the pieces through the salad just before serving.

PER SERVING

CALORIES	FAT	SAT FAT	CARBS	SUGARS	FIBRE	PROTEIN	SALT
331	11G	6G	17G	15G	3.1G	36G	2.5G

SPECIAL SAUSAGES & BUTTERNUT SQUASH SALAD

SERVES 4
PREP TIME 20 minutes
COOK TIME 25 minutes

500g (1lb 2oz) butternut squash,
   cut into 1–2cm (½–¾ inch) cubes
spray oil
1 teaspoon garlic granules
1 teaspoon smoked paprika
1 teaspoon dried oregano
8 reduced-fat pork sausages
1 tablespoon brown sauce
90g (3¼oz) bag of baby leaf salad
salt and pepper

FOR THE DRESSING
2 tablespoons balsamic vinegar
2 teaspoons wholegrain mustard
2 teaspoons honey
1 teaspoon olive oil

My husband introduced me to 'sausages and salad' as a meal when we first met, and I quickly realized what a great combo this is! These sausages are special because they have a coating of brown sauce with herbs and spices for an extra flavour boost, which is delicious alongside sweet roasted butternut squash, salad and a balsamic and wholegrain mustard dressing.

1   Preheat 1 air fryer drawer to 200°C (400°F).

2   Place the squash cubes in a large bowl, spray with oil and season with salt and pepper. Toss a few times to make sure they are lightly coated with oil. Put the squash cubes into the air fryer and cook for 25 minutes, tossing every 5 minutes to ensure even cooking.

3   Make the sausage seasoning by mixing the garlic granules, smoked paprika and oregano in a small bowl. Put the sausages on a dinner plate and spread the brown sauce over them, making sure each sausage has a light coating, then sprinkle over the seasoning mix.

4   Preheat the second air fryer drawer to 180°C (350°F). Put the sausages in this drawer, spray with a little oil and cook for 15 minutes.

5   While everything is cooking, make the dressing by combining all the ingredients in a small bowl, stirring thoroughly to ensure the honey is fully incorporated. Divide the salad leaves between 4 bowls.

6   Once the squash is cooked (it should be fork-tender, so double-check this, as you can cook it for a little longer if needed), scatter it over the salad leaves. Now place 2 sausages on each plate and drizzle the dressing over each serving.

PER SERVING

CALORIES	FAT	SAT FAT	CARBS	SUGARS	FIBRE	PROTEIN	SALT
314	15G	4.8G	22G	12G	5,8G	20G	1.8G

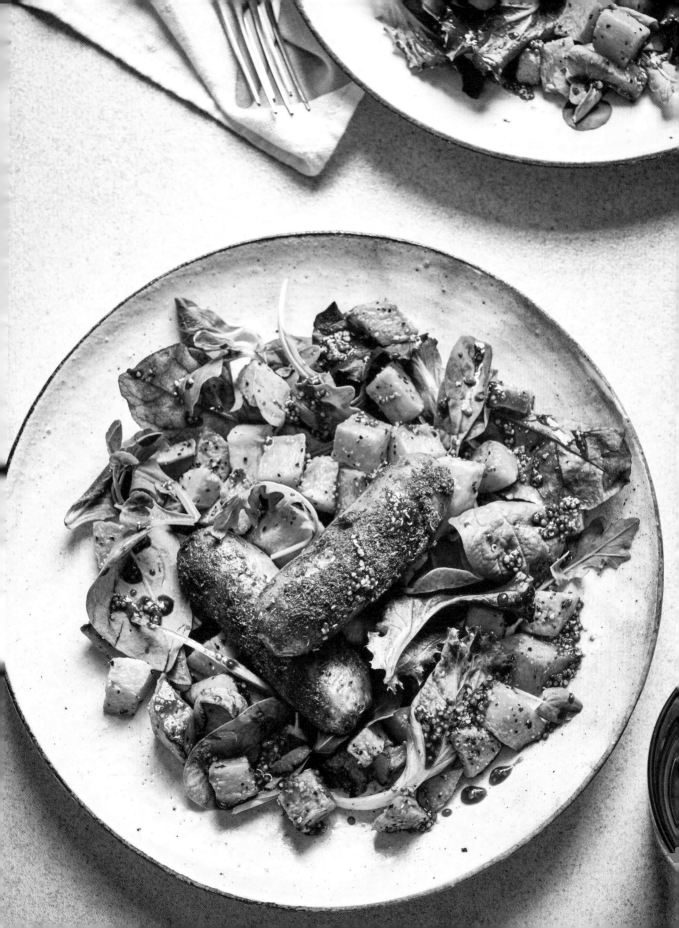

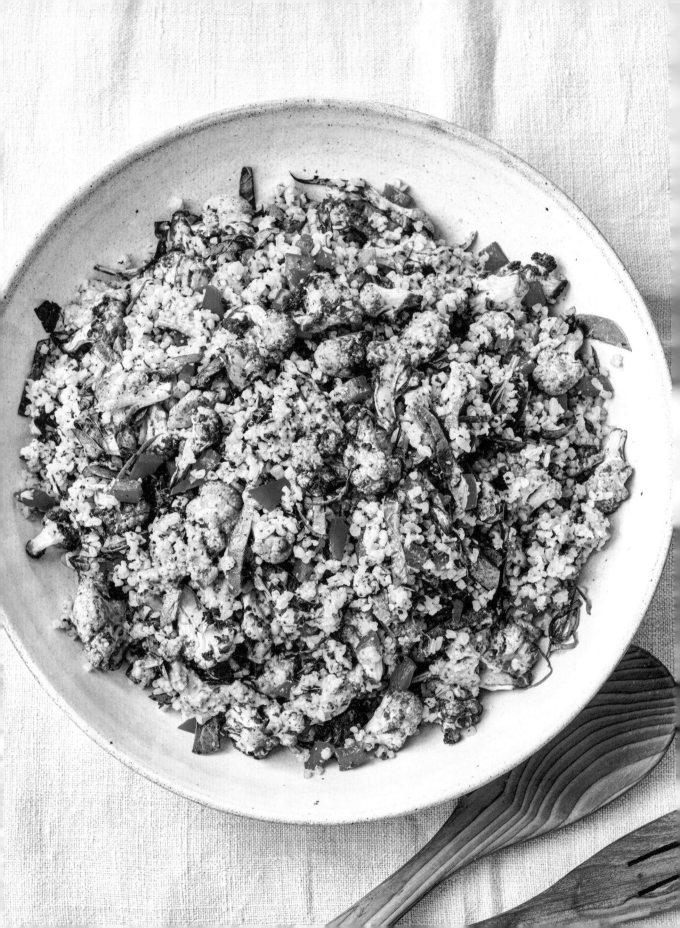

ROASTED CAULIFLOWER & PISTACHIO PESTO GRAIN SALAD

SERVES 4
PREP TIME 15 minutes
COOK TIME 25 minutes

200g (7oz) bulgur wheat

1 cauliflower, florets cut into bite-sized pieces, stalk sliced into thin batons

1 teaspoon sweet paprika

1 teaspoon garlic granules

½ teaspoon chilli powder

½ teaspoon coarsely ground salt

spray oil

2 large handfuls of baby spinach, shredded

1 red pepper, deseeded and finely chopped

FOR THE PISTACHIO PESTO

50g (1¾oz) shelled unsalted pistachios

2 handfuls of basil leaves, plus more (optional) to serve

1 handful of mint leaves, plus more (optional) to serve

45g (1¾oz) Parmesan-style vegetarian cheese, finely grated

juice of 1 lemon

1 teaspoon olive oil

½ teaspoon coarsely ground salt

Seasoned roasted cauliflower is combined with a lip-smacking pistachio pesto, mixed through bulgur wheat and red pepper. This is hearty, filling and delicious.

1 Cook the bulgur wheat on the hob according to the packet instructions, drain and leave to cool while you prepare the rest of the ingredients.

2 In a bowl, toss the cauliflower florets in the paprika, garlic granules, chilli powder and salt, then spray with oil. Toss again and spray with more oil. Repeat until all the cauliflower is lightly coated with oil.

3 Preheat both air fryer drawers to 200°C (400°F), divide the cauliflower equally between the 2 drawers and air fry for 8–10 minutes, until cooked and a little charred on the edges, but still with an al dente consistency.

4 Put all the pesto ingredients into a mini food processor and whizz until you have a mostly smooth paste. Ensure the nuts and cheese are well broken down, with no big lumps.

5 Place the cooked and cooled bulgur wheat in a large serving bowl, add the shredded spinach, chopped red pepper and cooked cauliflower, then stir through the pesto. Serve scattered with more herbs, if you like.

PER SERVING

CALORIES	FAT	SAT FAT	CARBS	SUGARS	FIBRE	PROTEIN	SALT
379	14G	3.6G	46G	6.2G	7.9G	15G	1.5G

RIGATONI ALLA NORMA

ROASTED RED PEPPER & ALMOND FETTUCINE

MARINARA SAUCE

CHEESY CHORIZO ORZO

LEMONY PRAWN & ASPARAGUS ORECCHIETTE

EASY CHEESY GARLIC MUSHROOM TAGLIATELLE

SUNDRIED TOMATO PASTA SALAD

ROAST GARLIC & TAHINI CAPELLINI WITH CRISPY CAVOLO NERO

RIBBONED COURGETTE MANFREDINE WITH GORGONZOLA

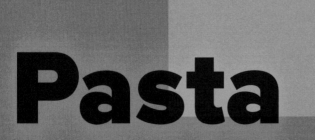

Pasta

RIGATONI ALLA NORMA

SERVES 4
PREP TIME 10 minutes
COOK TIME 20 minutes

2 aubergines (total weight about 500g / 1lb 2oz), chopped into 2cm (¾ inch) chunks

spray oil

350g (12oz) cherry tomatoes, or baby plum tomatoes, halved

360g (12½oz) rigatoni or rigatini pasta

4 garlic cloves, crushed

1 red chilli, deseeded and finely chopped

1 teaspoon olive oil

large handful of basil leaves, shredded

salt and pepper

Parmesan-style vegetarian cheese, finely grated, to serve

This take on the traditional Sicilian dish uses the power of the air fryer to roast the aubergine and tomatoes for the sauce. You can add in extras if you fancy: olives, capers, anchovies and sundried tomatoes would all give a lovely flavour boost. Serve with rocket drizzled with balsamic vinegar.

1 Remove the crisper plates and preheat both air fryer drawers to 200°C (400°F).

2 Place the aubergine chunks in a mixing bowl and spray with oil, tossing as you go to get good coverage. Divide equally between the 2 drawers, shake so they are in a single layer, and cook for 5 minutes.

3 Add the tomatoes, dividing them equally between the 2 drawers, reduce the temperature to 190°C (375°F) and cook for 15 minutes, stirring every 5 minutes.

4 Meanwhile, cook the pasta on the hob according to the packet instructions, (usually 10–12 minutes). When you drain it, reserve a little of the cooking water.

5 When there are 5 minutes remaining on the aubergine and tomatoes, add the garlic and chilli, again dividing them between the 2 drawers and stir well, squishing the tomatoes a little as you go. Cook for the final 5 minutes.

6 Stir the aubergine and tomato mixture through the pasta, add the olive oil, salt and pepper to taste, then add a little of the reserved pasta water to ensure the sauce is not too dry. Stir in the basil and serve with a tablespoon of grated cheese per person.

PER SERVING

CALORIES	FAT	SAT FAT	CARBS	SUGARS	FIBRE	PROTEIN	SALT
446	8.7G	3.5G	68G	8.9G	8.3G	19G	0.42G

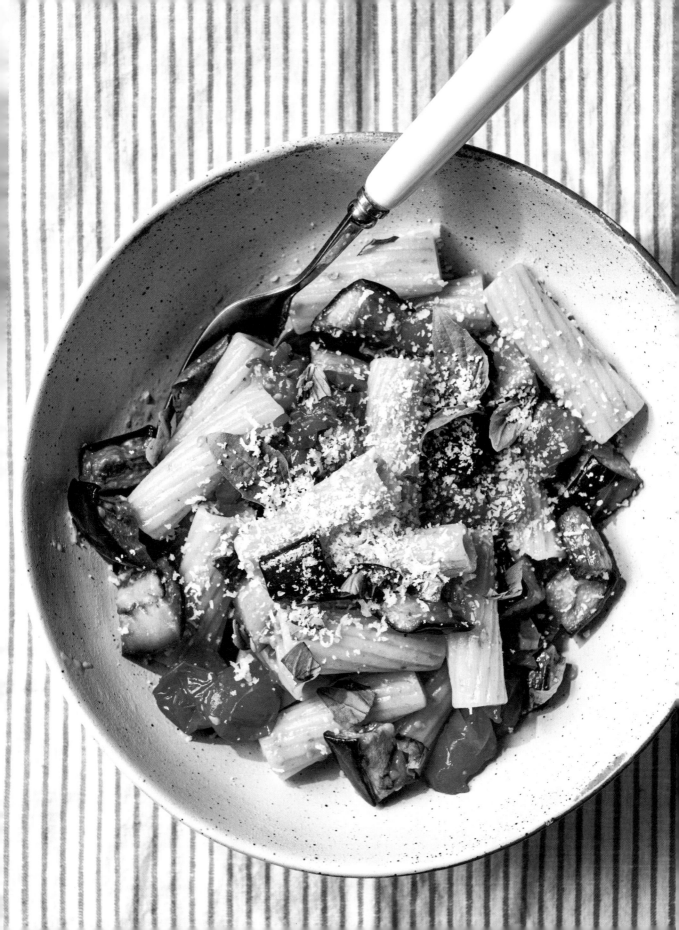

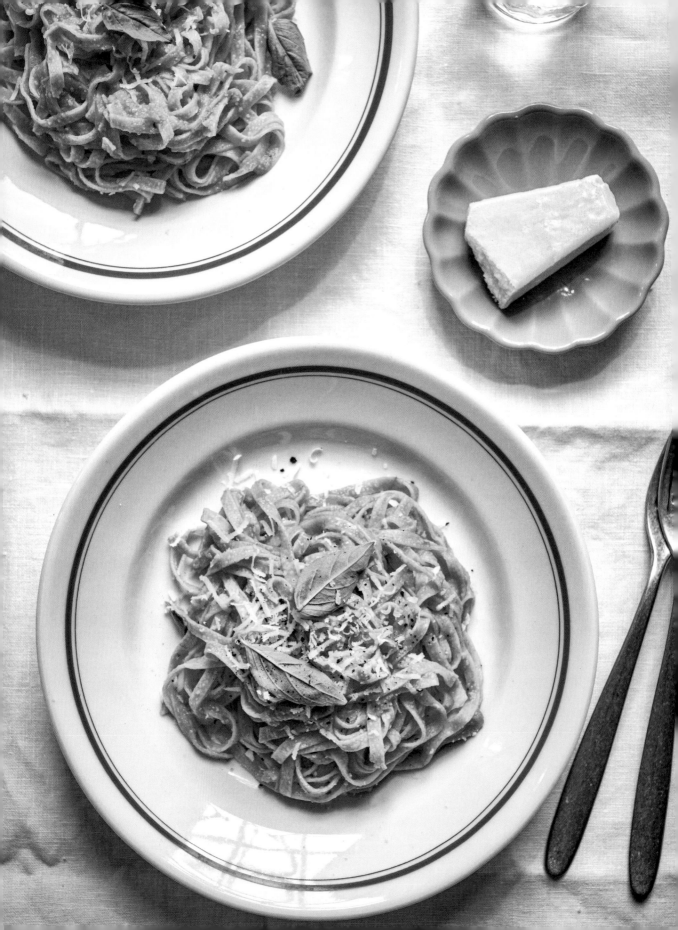

ROASTED RED PEPPER & ALMOND FETTUCINE

SERVES 4
PREP TIME 5 minutes
COOK TIME 15 minutes

4 red peppers

1 tablespoon olive oil

3 garlic cloves, each cut into
   3 pieces

50g (1¾oz) flaked almonds

360g (12½oz) fettucine, linguine,
   or spaghetti

1 teaspoon coarsely ground salt

a few basil leaves, plus more to
   serve

pinch of chilli flakes (optional)

Parmesan-style vegetarian cheese,
   finely grated, to serve

pepper

This is a simple pasta sauce which is perfect as an al fresco summer meal. The air fryer is great for roasting whole red peppers, and these are whizzed into a sauce with toasted almonds and garlic for a light and fresh pasta dish. Serve with a simple salad.

1 Preheat 1 air fryer drawer to 200°C (400°F). Prepare the red peppers by slicing off the tops as close to the stalk as possible and scooping out all the seeds (you want to keep the peppers whole). Place the peppers in the preheated drawer, cut sides down, and cook for 12 minutes.

2 Remove the crisper plate from the other air fryer drawer and preheat that drawer to 200°C (400°F). Put the olive oil and garlic pieces into an ovenproof ramekin. Place it in the preheated drawer, then spread the flaked almonds in an even layer over the bottom of the drawer around the ramekin. Cook for 5 minutes (check on the garlic and almonds after 4 minutes to ensure they are becoming golden and toasted but not burned).

3 After the peppers have cooked for 12 minutes, use silicone tongs to flip them over so they are cut side up, and cook them for another 3 minutes.

4 When everything is almost ready, cook the pasta on the hob according to the packet instructions.

5 Put the roasted peppers into a food processor or blender with the toasted almonds, garlic and its oil, salt, basil leaves and chilli, if using, and blend into a smooth sauce.

6 Drain the pasta, reserving a little of the cooking water, then stir in the sauce, adding a little bit of the reserved water to help make it smooth and silky.

7 Serve with grated cheese, torn basil leaves and black pepper.

PER SERVING

CALORIES	FAT	SAT FAT	CARBS	SUGARS	FIBRE	PROTEIN	SALT
538	17G	4.2G	70G	10G	9.3G	20G	1.5G

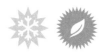

MARINARA SAUCE

SERVES 8
PREP TIME 5 minutes
COOK TIME 25 minutes

1kg (2lb 4oz) cherry tomatoes

6 garlic cloves, squashed with the flat edge of a knife so they flatten and burst slightly

1 small onion, finely chopped

1 tablespoon balsamic vinegar

1 teaspoon dried oregano

1 teaspoon honey

1 teaspoon coarsely ground salt

pepper

small handful of basil leaves

Roasting tomatoes in the air fryer adds a new dimension of flavour to this most basic of pasta sauces, which is always great to have on hand for easy meals of pasta or pizza. I always make a big batch of this sauce so I can keep some in the fridge or freezer for emergencies, but feel free to halve the recipe and cook it in just one air fryer drawer if you prefer.

1 Remove the crisper plates and preheat both air fryer drawers to 200°C (400°F).

2 Mix all the ingredients, apart from the basil, in a large mixing bowl, then divide equally between the air fryer drawers. Cook for 25 minutes, giving them a stir every 5 minutes.

3 Transfer to a food processor or blender, add the basil and whizz into a smooth sauce, or leave it chunky if you prefer.

4 Once cooled, store in glass jars or in an airtight plastic container in the refrigerator for up to 5 days.

PER SERVING

CALORIES	FAT	SAT FAT	CARBS	SUGARS	FIBRE	PROTEIN	SALT
48	0.7G	0.1G	6.4G	5.9G	2G	1.7G	0.63G

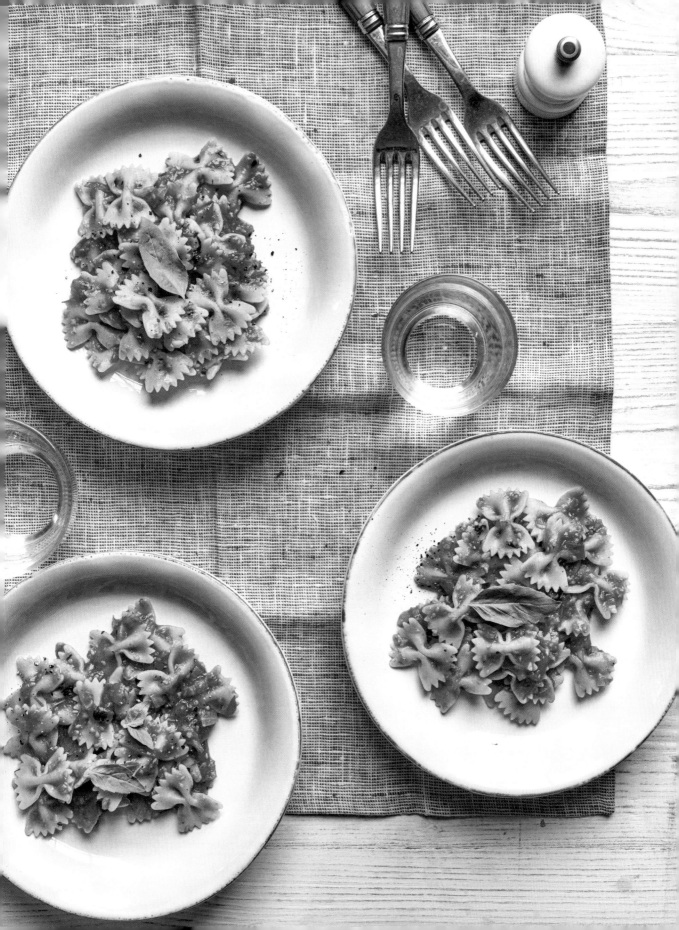

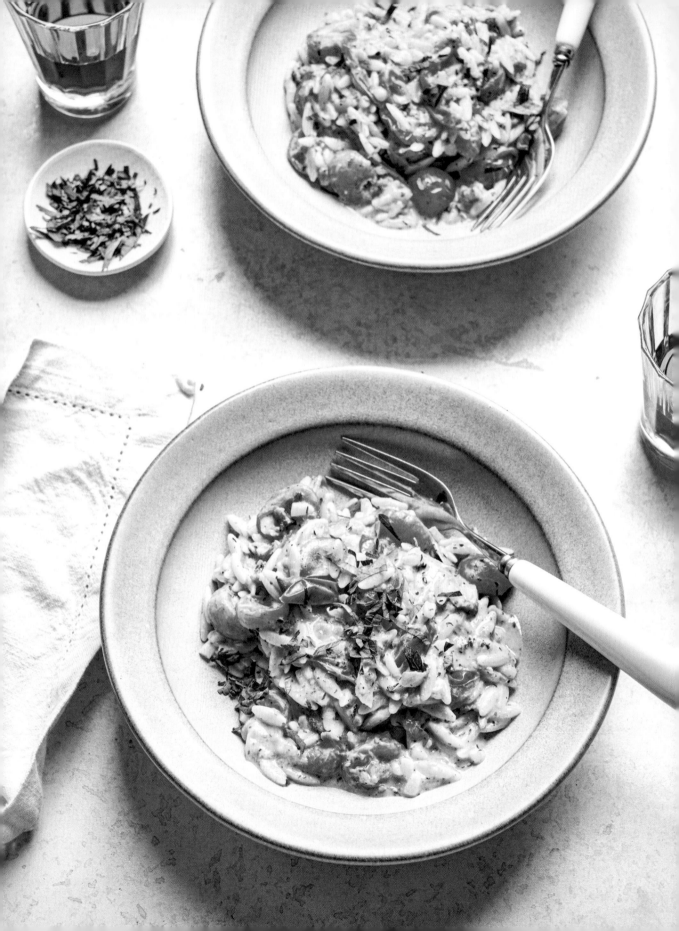

CHEESY CHORIZO ORZO

SERVES 4
PREP TIME 10 minutes
COOK TIME 16 minutes

50g (1¾oz) chorizo, finely chopped

1 onion, finely chopped

spray oil

250g (9oz) cherry tomatoes, halved

3 garlic cloves, crushed

2 teaspoons dried mixed herbs

½ teaspoon coarsely ground salt

½ teaspoon cracked black pepper

350g (12oz) orzo

1 litre (1¾ pints) hot chicken stock

120g (4¼oz) reduced-fat cream cheese

chopped parsley leaves, to serve

This has the smoky flavour of chorizo combined with creamy, cheesy orzo and herby tomatoes, which combine to make a comforting and satisfying meal which has long been a blog favourite. The air fryer brings out the best in both the chorizo and tomatoes in this dish. You can serve it with fresh green vegetables, such as asparagus or Tenderstem broccoli, on the side.

1 Remove the crisper plate from 1 of the air fryer drawers and preheat that drawer to 180°C (350°F).

2 Put the chorizo and onion into the drawer and spray with some oil. Cook for 8 minutes, stirring every few minutes.

3 Add the tomatoes, garlic, mixed herbs, salt and pepper and cook for another 8 minutes, stirring halfway through.

4 Meanwhile, cook the orzo in the hot stock on the hob following the packet instructions for the cooking time, as different brands can vary, but it is usually 7–9 minutes. Stir the orzo every now and again as it can stick to the pan. Drain the orzo over a bowl, reserving any liquid.

5 Add the cream cheese to the air fryer drawer, then the orzo with a little of its reserved cooking liquid and stir everything together to melt the cheese throughout the pasta. Add more pasta cooking water if needed.

6 Serve in warmed bowls, scattered with parsley.

PER SERVING

CALORIES	FAT	SAT FAT	CARBS	SUGARS	FIBRE	PROTEIN	SALT
497	9.5G	4.1G	72G	8G	4.7G	28G	2.1G

LEMONY PRAWN & ASPARAGUS ORECCHIETTE

SERVES 4
PREP TIME 10 minutes
COOK TIME 12 minutes

300g (10½oz) orecchiette pasta

240g (8½oz) large raw prawns, shelled

1 tablespoon olive oil

juice and finely grated zest of 1 lemon

1 teaspoon coarsely ground salt

½ teaspoon cracked black pepper

½ teaspoon garlic granules

180g (6oz) asparagus, sliced into 2–3cm (1 inch) pieces

4 garlic cloves, crushed

30g (1oz) Parmesan cheese, finely grated

handful of basil leaves, torn

A zesty, fresh pasta dish which is perfect for spring and summer. You can eat it as a stand-alone meal, or serve with extra seasonal green vegetables, salad or fresh bread.

1 Cook the pasta on the hob according to the packet instructions, (usually 10–12 minutes), reserving some of the pasta water when you drain it.

2 Meanwhile, place the prawns in a bowl and pat them dry with kitchen paper. Add ½ tablespoon of the olive oil, half the lemon zest and half the salt, along with the pepper and the garlic granules.

3 Preheat 1 air fryer drawer to 190°C (375°F), add the prawns in a single layer (allow a little space between each) and cook for 8 minutes; if your prawns are on the small side, reduce the time by a couple of minutes. Either way, shake halfway through.

4 Remove the crisper plate from the other air fryer drawer and preheat that drawer to 190°C (375°F). Add the asparagus and remaining ½ tablespoon of olive oil, stir to coat the asparagus and cook for 4 minutes. Add the crushed garlic, the remaining salt and lemon zest, stir and cook for another 2 minutes.

5 Add the cooked pasta to the drawer containing the asparagus, then tip in the cooked prawns, lemon juice, Parmesan and a splash of the pasta water, stir thoroughly, then stir in the basil. Divide between warmed bowls and serve.

PER SERVING

CALORIES	FAT	SAT FAT	CARBS	SUGARS	FIBRE	PROTEIN	SALT
383	7.6G	2.2G	53G	3.4G	4.6G	24G	1.7G

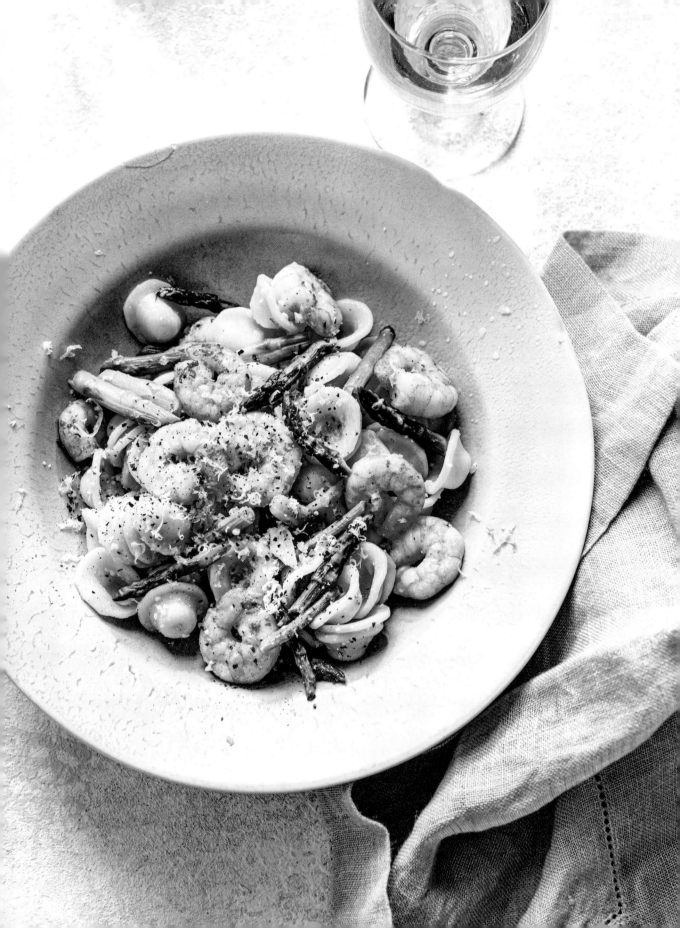

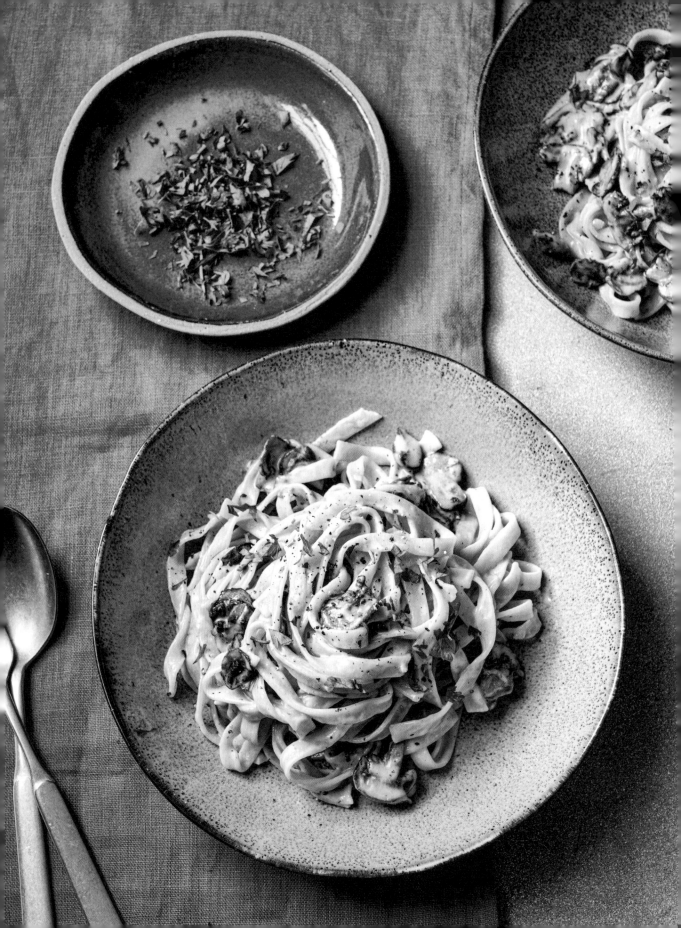

EASY CHEESY GARLIC MUSHROOM TAGLIATELLE

SERVES 4
PREP TIME 10 minutes
COOK TIME 12 minutes

300g (10½oz) tagliatelle

485g (1lb 1oz) chestnut mushrooms, sliced

spray oil

4 garlic cloves, crushed

1 green chilli, deseeded and finely chopped

150g reduced-fat cream cheese

200ml (7fl oz) hot vegetable stock

½ teaspoon coarsely ground salt

½ teaspoon cracked black peppercorns

handful of finely chopped parsley leaves

A simple but delicious pasta dish: creamy, mushroomy and garlicky... what more could you want? Air frying really helps to bring out the flavour of the mushrooms in this dish.

1   Remove the crisper plates and preheat both air fryer drawers to 180°C (350°F).

2   Cook tagliatelle on the hob according to the packet instructions, (usually 10–12 minutes).

3   Divide the mushrooms between the 2 drawers and spray with oil. Cook for 8 minutes, stirring halfway through.

4   Divide the garlic and chilli between the 2 drawers, stir into the mushrooms and cook for another 2 minutes.

5   Combine the mushrooms so that they are all in 1 drawer, then add the cream cheese and hot stock and stir well. Season with the salt and pepper.

6   Drain the pasta, reserving a little of the cooking water, and stir it through the garlic mushroom sauce. If it needs loosening, add some of the pasta water. Serve in bowls, scattered with parsley.

PER SERVING

CALORIES	FAT	SAT FAT	CARBS	SUGARS	FIBRE	PROTEIN	SALT
346	6.5G	3.1G	54G	5.3G	5.6G	15G	1.3G

SUNDRIED TOMATO PASTA SALAD

SERVES 4
PREP TIME 15 minutes
COOK TIME 45 minutes

1 red onion, finely chopped

juice of 1 lemon

300g (10½oz) farfalle

large handful of baby spinach, roughly chopped

small handful of basil leaves, roughly chopped

60g (2¼oz) Kalamata olives, sliced

20g (¾oz) sunflower seeds

FOR THE SUNDRIED TOMATOES

400g (14oz) cherry tomatoes, quartered (or halved if small)

1 tablespoon olive oil

2 teaspoons Italian seasoning

½ teaspoon coarsely ground salt

FOR THE DRESSING

juice of 1 lemon

1 teaspoon Dijon mustard

1 garlic clove, crushed

1 teaspoon honey

1 teaspoon olive oil

salt and pepper

The air fryer makes brilliant sundried tomatoes which provide intense bursts of flavour in this Mediterranean-inspired salad.

1 First prepare the tomatoes by placing them in a mixing bowl with the olive oil, Italian seasoning and salt.

2 Preheat both air fryer drawers to 120°C (250°F). Divide the tomatoes equally between the 2 drawers, spread into a single layer, and cook for 45 minutes, shaking a few times during the cooking time. (Please note that if you are using some types of air fryer, you will need to select the 'roast' function to be able to set the required low temperature – consult the manufacturer's instructions.)

3 For the salad, place the onion in a small bowl with the lemon juice.

4 Cook the pasta on the hob according to the packet instructions, (usually 10–12 minutes), then drain and rinse under cold water to prevent it cooking any further or sticking together.

5 To make the dressing, whisk together the lemon juice, mustard, garlic, honey and olive oil and season with salt and pepper (or place all the ingredients in a jam jar and give it a good shake).

6 Once the tomatoes are ready, they should be dried, but still pliable and not burnt.

7 Put the cooked pasta into a large bowl with the spinach, most of the basil, the red onion in its lemon juice and the olives. Add the roasted tomatoes, then the dressing. Toss well to combine, then scatter over the sunflower seeds and remaining basil leaves before serving.

PER SERVING

CALORIES	FAT	SAT FAT	CARBS	SUGARS	FIBRE	PROTEIN	SALT
448	13G	1.8G	65G	13G	6.7G	13G	1.7G

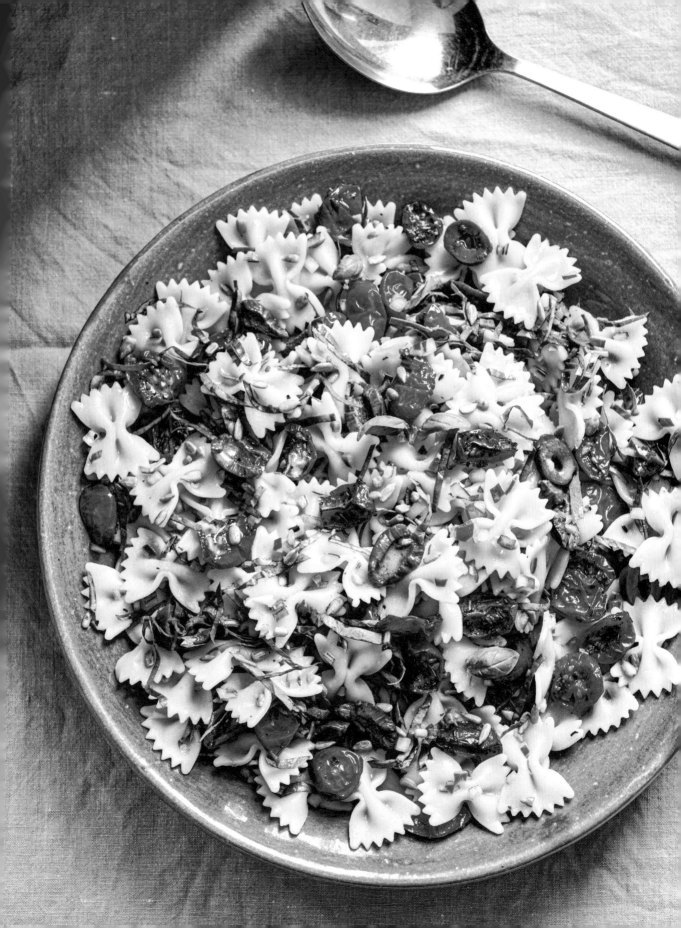

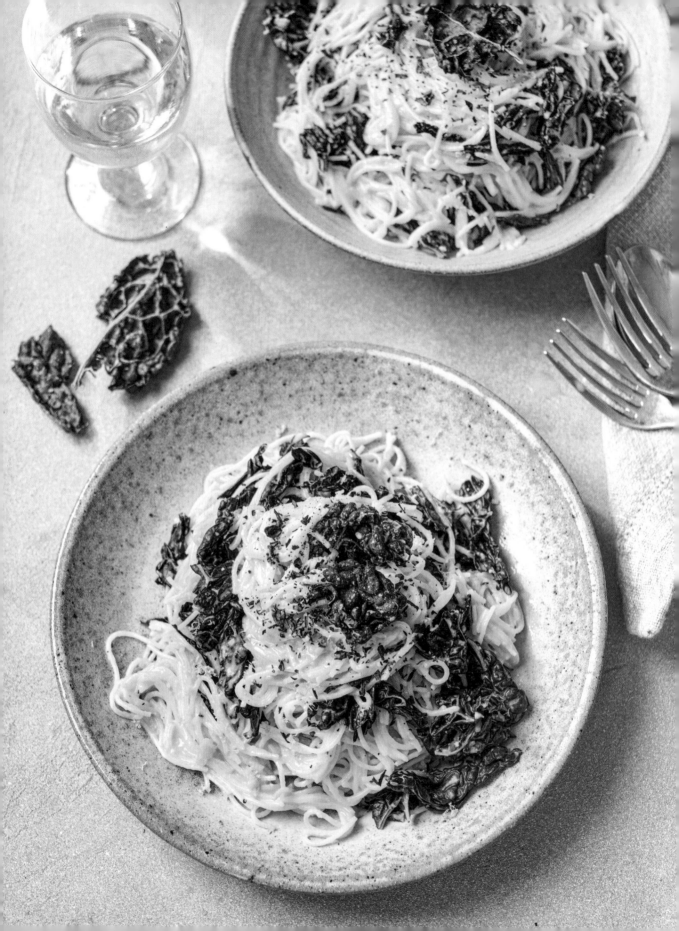

ROAST GARLIC & TAHINI CAPELLINI WITH CRISPY CAVOLO NERO

SERVES 2
PREP TIME 5 minutes
COOK TIME 30 minutes

1 garlic bulb
juice and finely grated zest of
    2 lemons
2 tablespoons tahini
2 teaspoons olive oil
400g (14oz) cavolo nero
160g (5¾oz) capellini
salt

The lemony sauce in this dish utilizes a whole head of roast garlic, which is ridiculously easy to make in the air fryer, where it develops a mellow flavour. I use capellini pasta here which is essentially thin spaghetti that provides lots of surface area for this tasty sauce to cling to. Angel hair spaghetti or vermicelli would work brilliantly too. The quantity of cavolo nero might seem a lot, but it shrinks almost to nothing when it's cooked.

1 First roast the garlic. Slice off the top of the bulb so that all the cloves are exposed. Brush some olive oil over the cut garlic and add a pinch of salt. Wrap the bulb in foil. Preheat 1 air fryer drawer to 200°C (400°F), then cook the garlic for 25 minutes.

2 Let the garlic parcel cool for about 10 minutes before squeezing the garlic from its cloves into a small bowl. Add the lemon zest and juice, the tahini, 1 teaspoon of the olive oil and some salt. Stir well, slightly squishing the garlic into the paste, but it's fine to have some whole cloves left in there too.

3 Preheat both air fryer drawers to 200°C (400°F).

4 Prepare the cavolo nero by removing the stalks and tearing the leaves into bite-sized pieces. Place in a bowl with 1 tablespoon of the garlic-tahini mix and the remaining 1 teaspoon olive oil, then massage into the leaves. Divide between the 2 air fryer drawers and cook for 4–6 minutes, giving the drawers a shake halfway through. Some leaves will be crispy and some will be moist, but it's nice to have a mix of both. Set aside.

5 Cook the pasta on the hob according to the packet instructions, reserving some of the cooking water when you drain it. Add a couple of tablespoons of pasta water to the garlic-tahini paste to loosen it, then add to the pasta and stir thoroughly, adding a little more pasta water if it needs it.

6 Add the cavolo nero and stir it through, then serve.

PER SERVING

CALORIES	FAT	SAT FAT	CARBS	SUGARS	FIBRE	PROTEIN	SALT
520	17.7G	2.5G	58.9G	6.3G	13.3G	20.7G	0.5G

RIBBONED COURGETTE MANFREDINE WITH GORGONZOLA

SERVES 2
PREP TIME 10 minutes
COOK TIME 12 minutes

This frilly-edged pasta looks especially pretty with ribboned courgettes, which similarly crinkle as they cook. But feel free to serve this sauce with any other long, flat pasta shape.

2 large courgettes (or 4 small)

1 garlic clove, finely grated

2 teaspoons olive oil

finely grated zest of 1 lemon

60g (2¼oz) Gorgonzola cheese, crumbled

200g (7oz) manfredine, to serve (or see recipe introduction)

salt and pepper

1 Prepare the courgettes by halving them lengthways, then ribboning them with a vegetable peeler straight into a bowl (you could also chop long fine pieces with a knife). Mix the garlic and olive oil with the lemon zest and some salt to season, then add to the courgettes and toss until everything is coated.

2 Preheat both air fryer drawers to 160°C (325°F). Divide the courgettes between the 2 drawers and cook for 10 minutes, stirring halfway through. When the courgettes are cooked and crisped at the edges, tip them into a bowl and stir through most of the Gorgonzola until it melts.

3 Cook the pasta on the hob according to the packet instructions, then drain, reserving some of the cooking water. Stir the cheesy courgettes through the pasta, adding a little water if needed, then top with the remaining Gorgonzola and season with pepper to serve.

PER SERVING

CALORIES	FAT	SAT FAT	CARBS	SUGARS	FIBRE	PROTEIN	SALT
536	15G	6.5G	74G	9G	6.2G	22G	1.3G

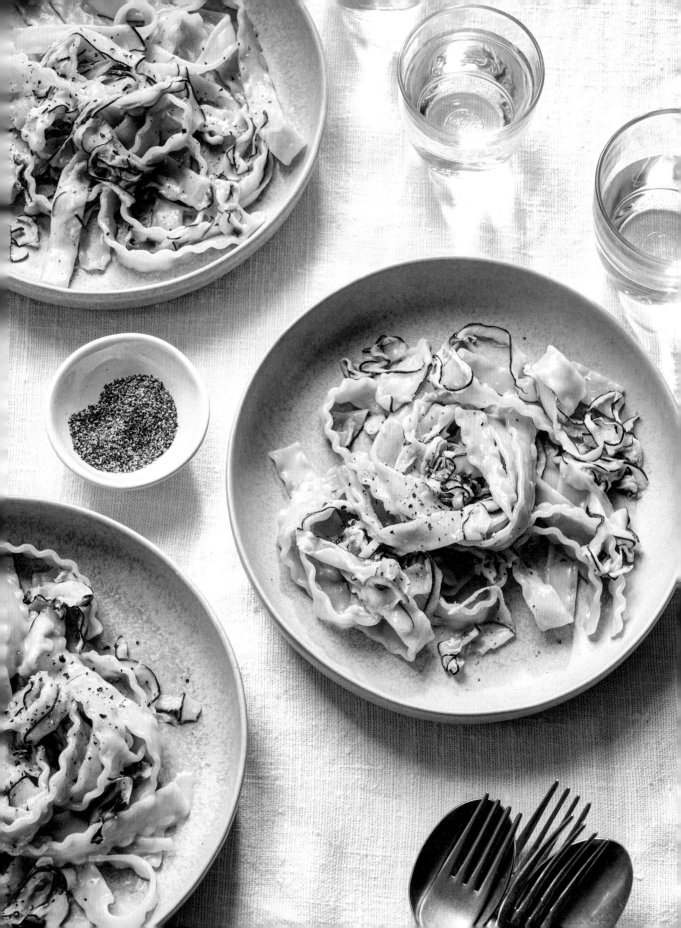

WHOLE TANDOORI ROAST
CHICKEN

SUMAC CHICKEN COUSCOUS

HARISSA & HERB MOROCCAN-
STYLE MEATBALLS

HUNTER'S CHICKEN

ITALIAN-STYLE MOZZARELLA
STUFFED BURGERS

CHAR SIU PORK

PRAWN & CHORIZO PAELLA

WORCESTERSHIRE ROAST
BEEF

CURRIED CHICKEN RISSOLES

HONEY BARBECUE
HEDGEHOG CHICKEN

PERFECT STEAK

ROCKET PESTO STUFFED
TOMATOES

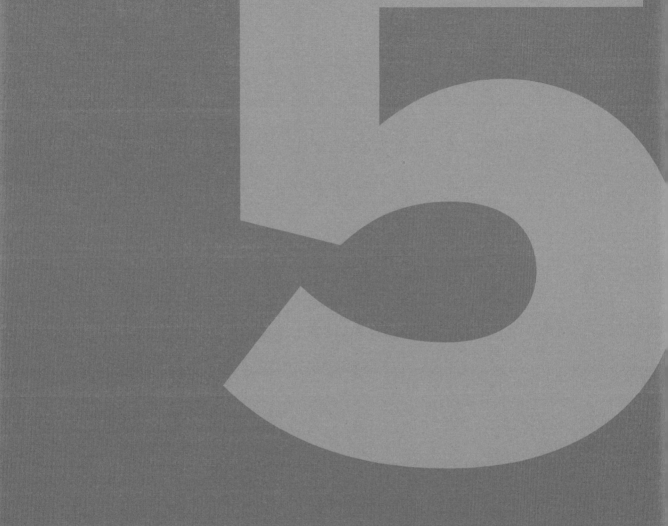

5

Family favourites

WHOLE TANDOORI ROAST CHICKEN

SERVES 4–6
PREP TIME 5 minutes, plus marinating
COOK TIME 1 hour

1 whole chicken, about 1.6kg (3lb 8oz), make sure it will fit into your air fryer drawer
1 tablespoon mild tandoori spice mix
1 teaspoon fat-free Greek yogurt
1 teaspoon red wine vinegar
salt and pepper

A whole chicken is quicker to cook in the air fryer than the oven, and this tandoori spiced chicken has long been a blog favourite! If you can marinate it in advance, or even overnight, you will get enhanced flavour, but if you only have time to throw it together right before you cook the chicken, you'll still have a tasty meal to pair perfectly with chips, Bombay potatoes or rice. It also works as a lunchtime filling for pittas or wraps.

1   Make sure you take your chicken out of the refrigerator about 1 hour before cooking it.

2   In a small bowl, combine the tandoori spice mix, Greek yogurt and vinegar, then add some salt and pepper. Mix to form the tandoori marinade. Use your fingers to loosen the chicken skin over the breast, then cover the whole chicken in the marinade, including underneath the breast skin. Leave to marinate while it comes up to room temperature (or you can do this the night before cooking, if you prefer and have time).

3   Preheat 1 air fryer drawer to 180°C (350°F).

4   Place the chicken breast side down in the air fryer drawer and press it down. Cook for 1 hour, turning it halfway through. Make sure there are no bits of the chicken sticking up above the edge of the air fryer drawer, as you do not want it coming into contact with the heating element.

5   Check the chicken is completely cooked; the internal temperature should be at least 75°C (167°F). Alternatively, insert the point of a knife into into the breast to ensure the juices run clear. Allow to rest for 15 minutes before carving.

PER SERVING (IF FOR 4 – INCLUDES SKIN)

CALORIES	FAT	SAT FAT	CARBS	SUGARS	FIBRE	PROTEIN	SALT
534	36G	10G	1.6G	0.7G	0.6G	50G	1.1G

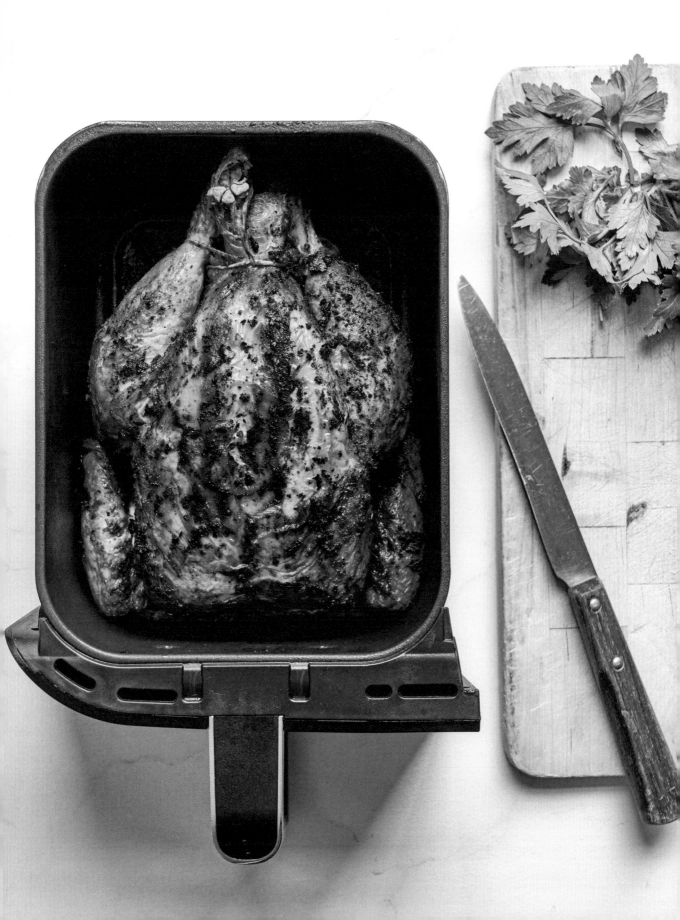

SUMAC CHICKEN COUSCOUS

SERVES 4
PREP TIME 15 minutes
COOK TIME 20 minutes

---

2 skinless chicken breast fillets

2 tablespoons sumac

spray oil

1 red onion, finely chopped

1 head of broccoli, florets
    separated, stalk trimmed
    and grated

200g (7oz) couscous

250ml (9fl oz) hot chicken stock

juice and finely grated zest of
    1 lime

1 tablespoon honey

1 tablespoon red wine vinegar

handful of parsley leaves, finely
    chopped

handful of mint leaves, finely
    chopped

1 carrot, grated

salt and pepper

Simple zesty, fresh flavours guaranteed that this meal was a hit with my daughters. You can always toss in any extra veggies that you fancy, such as halved cherry tomatoes (air fry them with the broccoli if you want to soften them up), chopped cucumber, green beans, peas and so on. I just stick to the vegetables that I know my children will eat without a fuss!

1   Remove the crisper plate from 1 air fryer drawer and heat that drawer to 180°C (350°F).

2   Place the chicken in a bowl and sprinkle with 1 tablespoon of the sumac, tossing to coat, then spray with oil. Place the chicken in the air fryer and cook for 20 minutes. Halfway through the cooking time, turn the chicken and add the red onion, spray with oil again and continue to cook, stirring the onion 5 minutes into its cooking time.

3   Preheat the second air fryer drawer to 180°C (350°F) with the crisper plate in, then add the broccoli florets. Spray with oil and cook for 9 minutes, shaking well halfway through cooking.

4   Put the couscous in a large bowl, pour over the hot stock, cover with a plate and leave for 5 minutes. Stir through the lime zest and juice, honey, vinegar, parsley, mint, salt and pepper, then add the grated broccoli and carrot.

5   Remove the chicken from the air fryer (check it is completely cooked; the internal temperature should be at least 75°C / 167°F), and thinly slice it. Stir the chicken, red onion and broccoli florets through the couscous, along with the remaining tablespoon of sumac, then serve.

PER SERVING

CALORIES	FAT	SAT FAT	CARBS	SUGARS	FIBRE	PROTEIN	SALT
366	3.2G	0.7G	47G	9.4G	9.5G	32G	0.7G

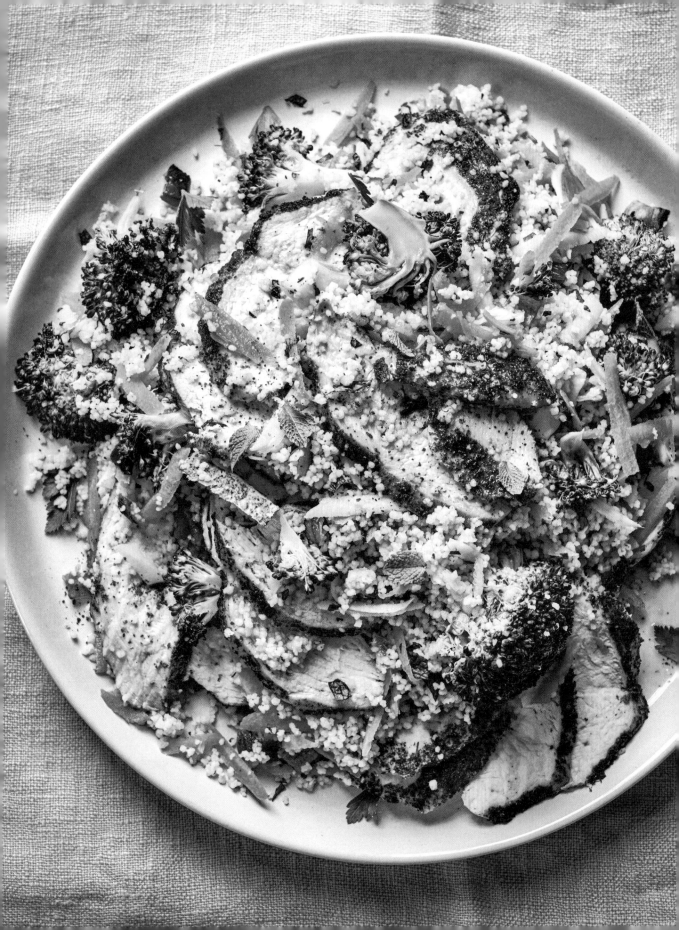

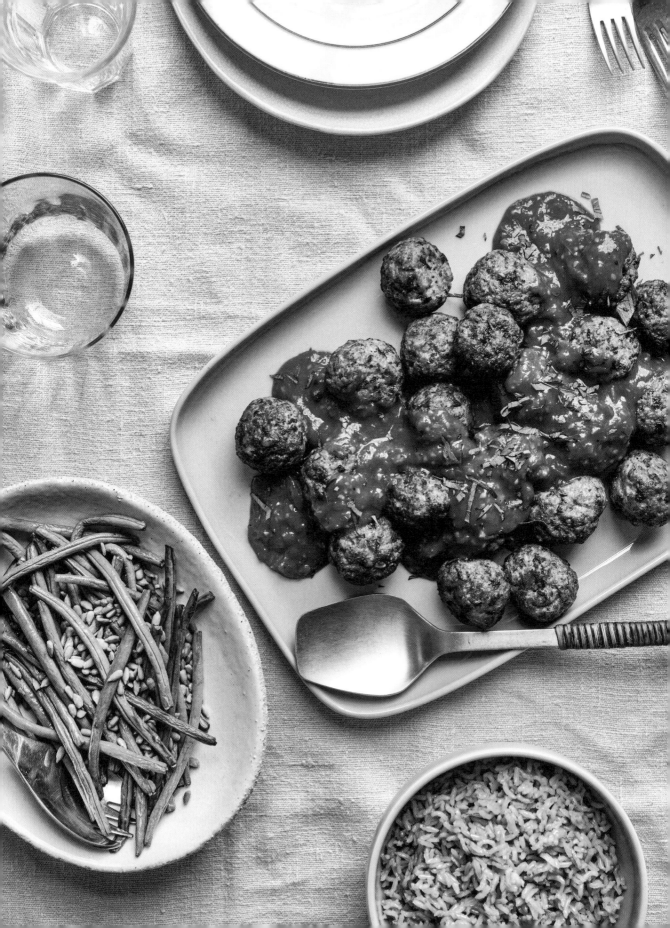

HARISSA & HERB MOROCCAN-STYLE MEATBALLS

SERVES 4
PREP TIME 15 minutes
COOK TIME 25 minutes

2 garlic cloves

handful of mint leaves

handful of parsley leaves and stalks

2 slices of wholemeal bread, roughly torn

500g (1lb 2oz) reduced-fat minced lamb (10 per cent fat)

1 egg, lightly beaten

FOR THE SAUCE

500g (1lb 2oz) cherry tomatoes

5 garlic cloves, each chopped into 2–3 pieces

1 green chilli, deseeded

1 tablespoon harissa paste

2 teaspoons honey

handful of parsley leaves and stalks, plus more (optional) to serve

handful of basil leaves, plus more (optional) to serve

salt and pepper

TO SERVE

200g (7oz) fine green beans, topped and tailed

spray oil

2 tablespoons sunflower seeds

500g (1lb 2oz) cooked brown rice

The delicious combination of roasted tomatoes and garlic, smoky harissa and herbs makes the perfect sauce for these meatballs. If you want to reduce the spiciness, leave out the green chilli and be cautious with the harissa (different brands can vary in heat). If you prefer, you can swap out the minced lamb for beef, chicken, turkey or pork, but give the meatballs a little spray of oil if you do this.

1   Remove the crisper plate from 1 of the air fryer drawers. Preheat both drawers to 180°C (350°F).

2   Make the meatballs by putting the garlic, herbs and bread into a food processor or blender and whizzing into fine crumbs. Add the lamb and egg and pulse-blend to thoroughly combine the ingredients, without turning the mixture into a paste. Roll into 22 equal-sized balls, each about 3cm (1¼ inches) in diameter.

3   Put all the sauce ingredients, apart from the herbs, into the drawer without the crisper plate, season well and stir with a silicone spatula. Cook for 20 minutes, stirring every 5 minutes.

4   Put half the meatballs in the other drawer, leaving a little space between each (you need to cook these in 2 batches to ensure the drawer is not overcrowded) and cook for 10 minutes, shaking halfway through cooking. Set the first batch aside and cover with foil to keep warm while you cook the second batch in the same way.

5   Once the sauce is cooked, use a silicone spatula to scrape it all into a food processor or blender, add the parsley and basil and purée into a smooth sauce (a stick blender can be used if you prefer).

6   Rinse or wipe out the sauce drawer with some kitchen paper (be careful if it is still hot) and add the green beans. Spray with oil, toss and add the sunflower seeds. Cook for 5 minutes at 180°C (350°F).

7   Stir the meatballs into the tomato sauce. Divide the rice between warmed bowls, top with meatballs and sauce and serve the green beans and sunflower seeds on the side. Scatter a few more fresh herbs over, if you have some, then serve.

PER SERVING

CALORIES	FAT	SAT FAT	CARBS	SUGARS	FIBRE	PROTEIN	SALT
503	17G	6.3G	48G	4.9G	6.5G	35G	0.64G

HUNTER'S CHICKEN

SERVES 4
PREP TIME 15 minutes
COOK TIME 45 minutes

---

4 skinless chicken breast fillets,
    each 150g (5½oz)
8 bacon medallions
120g (4¼oz) Cheddar cheese,
    grated
2 teaspoons mixed herbs
spray oil

FOR THE BARBECUE SAUCE
2 onions, finely chopped
2 teaspoons olive oil
250ml (9fl oz) tomato passata
2 tablespoons balsamic vinegar
2 tablespoons Worcestershire
    sauce
2 teaspoons honey
1 teaspoon chilli powder
    (optional)

A chicken breast smothered in barbecue sauce, bacon and cheese is always a hit in our house. I make my own sauce for this, but you can use a shop-bought barbecue sauce if you are short of time; just be aware that shop-bought sauces may have a high sugar content. I serve this with Southwestern corn salad (see page 151), but it goes equally well with fries (regular or sweet potato), rice or couscous, and any vegetables you fancy.

1 To make the barbecue sauce, heat the oil in a saucepan on the hob then fry the onions for 8 minutes. Stir in the remaining sauce ingredients and simmer for 10 minutes, until thickened.

2 Preheat both air fryer drawers to 180°C (350°F).

3 Butterfly the chicken breasts by slicing horizontally through the middle with a sharp knife, then opening each up. Add 2 teaspoons of sauce to the middle of each chicken breast, fold it back over, then wrap 2 bacon medallions around the opening of each chicken breast: they won't fully wrap around the whole breast but should cover the opening, so just wrap them around as best as you can.

4 Either use 2 silicone liners or 2 baking dishes that fit into your air fryer drawers, or fashion 2 foil dishes with sides about 2cm (1 inch) high. Place 2 chicken breasts side by side in each liner or dish. Sit them in the air fryer drawers and cook for 17 minutes.

5 Next, spoon the remaining barbecue sauce over the chicken, cover evenly with grated cheese and sprinkle over the mixed herbs. Spray with oil.

6 Increase the temperature of both air fryer drawers to 200°C (400°F) and cook for a further 8 minutes. By now the cheese should be golden brown and bubbling and the chicken cooked through. Check the chicken is completely cooked through; the internal temperature should be at least 75°C (167°F). Serve with your chosen accompaniments.

PER SERVING

CALORIES	FAT	SAT FAT	CARBS	SUGARS	FIBRE	PROTEIN	SALT
477	18G	7.9G	16G	14G	2.5G	61G	3.5G

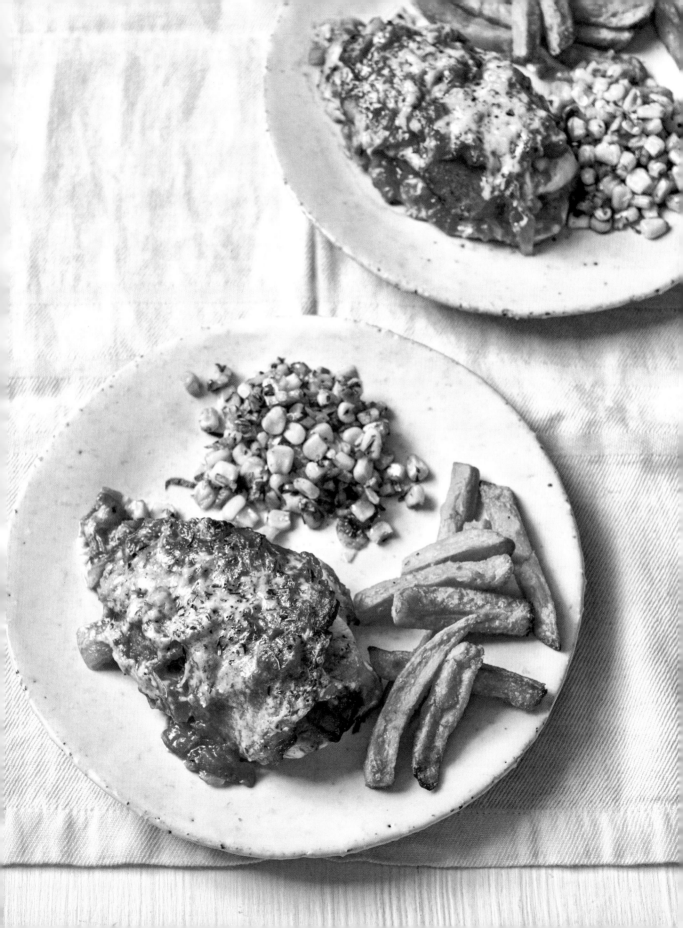

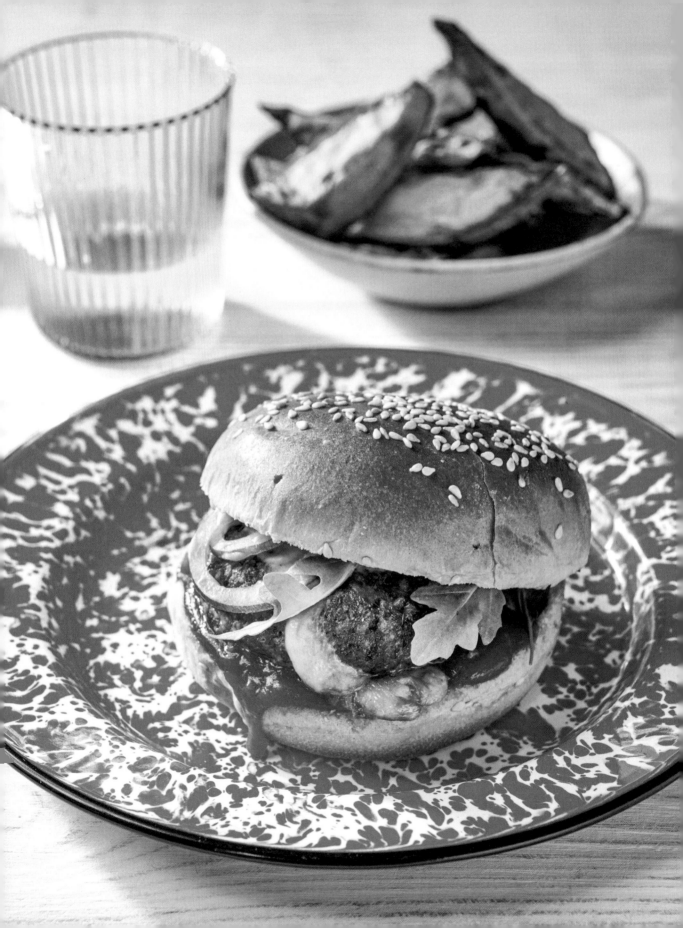

ITALIAN-STYLE MOZZARELLA STUFFED BURGERS

SERVES 4–6
PREP TIME 20 minutes, plus chilling
COOK TIME 17 minutes

50g (1¾oz) couscous

500g (1lb 2oz) 5 per cent fat minced beef

2 tablespoons tomato purée

1 teaspoon Dijon mustard

1 teaspoon Worcestershire sauce

1 teaspoon garlic granules

1 teaspoon onion granules

1 teaspoon Italian herbs

1 teaspoon salt

1 egg

150g (5½oz) pizza mozzarella (the firm variety that comes in a block), cut into 6 chunks of 25g (1oz) each

4–6 burger buns (I use brioche buns)

FOR THE FIXINGS (ALL OPTIONAL)
rocket
tomato slices
mustard
ketchup
sliced cheese

A tasty burger filled with oozing mozzarella: what could be better? I use couscous in these as a breadcrumb alternative to give them a lighter texture, and serve them with everyone's favourite fillings, usually alongside some fries or wedges and salad. These burgers are also great served as giant meatballs over a bowl of garlicky tomato spaghetti (try it with Marinara sauce, see page 74) and rocket! (You can freeze leftovers.)

1 Prepare the couscous by putting it in a small bowl and pouring over boiling water to just cover. Set aside, covered with a plate, and leave for 5 minutes.

2 In a large bowl, mix together the minced beef, tomato purée, mustard, Worcestershire sauce, garlic and onion granules, Italian herbs and salt. Add the cooked couscous and stir it in, then crack in the egg and stir that in thoroughly.

3 To make equal-sized burgers, weigh the mixture, divide the weight by 6 and make each burger that weight – around 120g (4¼oz) each. You can just do this by eye if you prefer! Use your hands to roll each piece into a large ball, then press a chunk of mozzarella into the middle and fully surround it with the meat mixture so it stays in the middle and doesn't leak out. Use your hands to press the balls into burger shapes roughly the size of the buns, allowing for a little shrinkage. Place on a plate, cover with clingfilm or an upturned dinner plate and chill for 30 minutes.

4 Once the burgers have chilled, preheat both air fryer drawers to 180°C (350°F). Place 2 burgers in each drawer and cook for 15 minutes – you can either cook the remaining 2 burgers in a second batch or freeze them for another day.

5 Cut the burger buns in half, remove the cooked burgers from the air fryer drawers and toast the burger buns (cut side up) for 2 minutes.

6 Assemble the burgers in the buns, adding any fixings that you fancy.

PER SERVING (NOT INCLUDING FIXINGS)

CALORIES	FAT	SAT FAT	CARBS	SUGARS	FIBRE	PROTEIN	SALT
524	19G	9.2G	43G	6.8G	2.6G	45G	2.8G

CHAR SIU PORK

SERVES 4
PREP TIME 10 minutes, plus marinating time
COOK TIME 25 minutes

It's no wonder that this has long been a favourite recipe on the blog: it works so perfectly in an air fryer, giving you that all-over slight char on the outside and tender pork in the middle. I usually serve it sliced up with egg-fried rice and edamame, baby corn or broccoli.

1 pork tenderloin fillet (450–500g / 1lb–1lb 2oz)
spray oil

FOR THE MARINADE
2 tablespoons tomato purée
2 tablespoons light soy sauce
1 tablespoon Chinese rice wine
1 tablespoon hoisin sauce
1 tablespoon honey
1 teaspoon Chinese 5 spice
1 teaspoon red food colouring (optional)

1   Make up the marinade in a bowl by mixing everything together. I like to add red food colouring as it does give the pork a more dramatic appearance, but you can leave it out if you prefer.

2   Cut the pork tenderloin in half, so it will fit in the air fryer drawer, then pop it into the bowl of marinade. Toss it around a bit to cover, then leave to marinate for at least 30 minutes. If you can leave it in the refrigerator overnight, even better!

3   Preheat 1 air fryer drawer to 180°C (350°F).

4   Spray a little oil into the drawer, add the 2 pork pieces, then spray them with oil. Cook for 25 minutes, turning halfway through. The pork should be caramelized and slightly charred on the outside and cooked through in the middle. You can check that it's done with a food thermometer: the internal temperature should be at least 75°C (167°F). Let the pork rest for 10 minutes before thinly slicing and serving.

PER SERVING

CALORIES	FAT	SAT FAT	CARBS	SUGARS	FIBRE	PROTEIN	SALT
247	4.3G	1.8G	10G	8.9G	1.5G	40G	1.2G

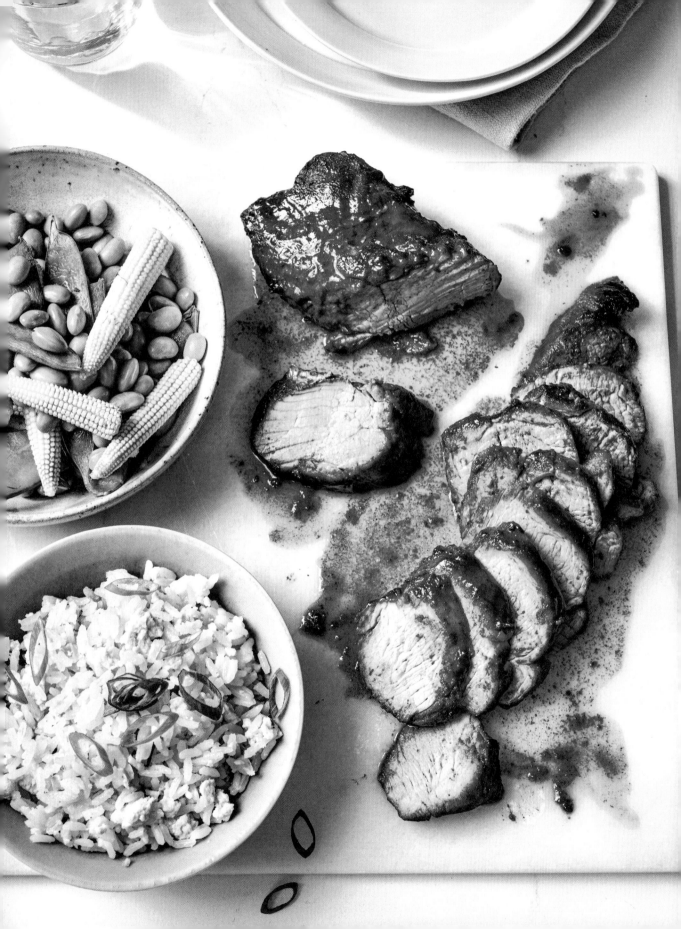

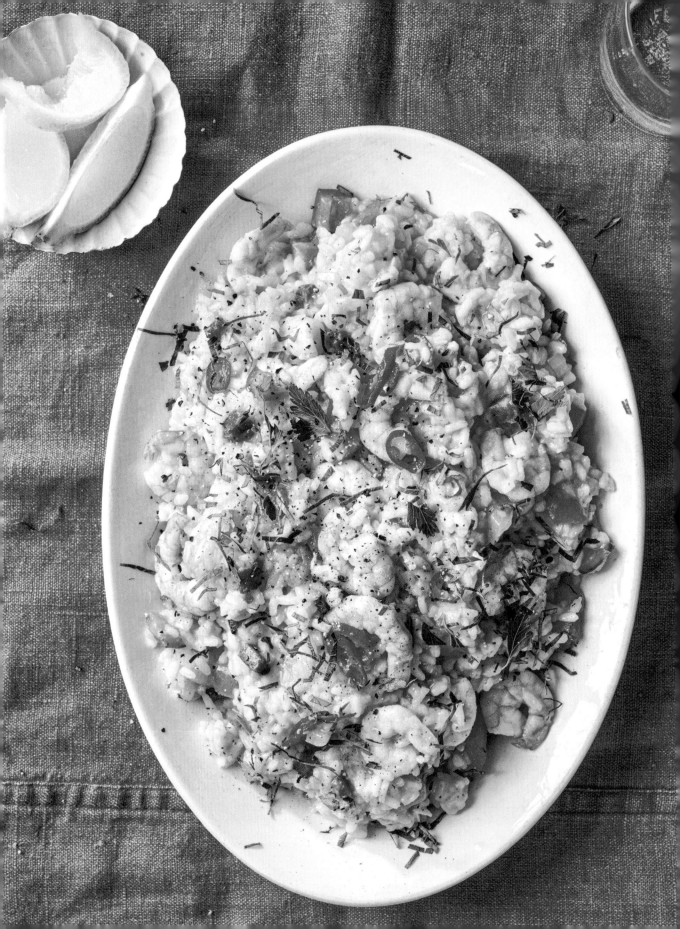

PRAWN & CHORIZO PAELLA

SERVES 4
PREP TIME 15 minutes
COOK TIME 25 minutes

3 teaspoons olive oil

300g (10½oz) paella rice

1 litre (1¾ pints) hot chicken stock
(you might not use it all)

pinch of saffron strands

½ teaspoon smoked paprika

80g (2¾oz) chorizo, finely
chopped

1 onion, finely chopped

2 red peppers, deseeded and finely
chopped

240g (8½oz) raw king prawns,
patted dry with kitchen paper

4 garlic cloves, crushed

1 red chilli, deseeded and finely
chopped

handful of parsley leaves, finely
chopped

salt and pepper

1 lemon, cut into 4 wedges,
to serve

A paella-style dish packed full of summery flavour, that should evoke holiday vibes with every bite! Chorizo works beautifully in the air fryer. I would usually serve this up with some extra vegetables, such as asparagus, fine green beans or sugarsnap peas. If you'd rather it weren't spicy, leave out the red chilli and make sure you don't buy spicy chorizo.

1   In a large saucepan over the hob, heat up 1 teaspoon of olive oil until it's sizzling, then stir in the paella rice for 1 minute. Pour in about 600ml (20fl oz) of the hot stock and bring the rice up to a fast simmer. Add the saffron and smoked paprika. The rice will need to cook for 20–25 minutes, at a simmer. Stir regularly to prevent it sticking to the bottom of the pan and top up with more stock if it has absorbed all the liquid.

2   Remove the crisper plates and preheat both air fryer drawers to 200°C (400°F).

3   Put the chorizo in the first drawer with the onion and peppers, and drizzle with 1 teaspoon more of the olive oil. Cook for 12 minutes, stirring a couple of times while cooking.

4   In the second drawer, arrange the prawns in a single layer, drizzling them with the remaining teaspoon of oil. Air fry for 8 minutes, stirring halfway through. For the final 2 minutes of cooking time, add the garlic and chilli to the prawns, stirring again as you do so.

5   Once the rice is cooked (taste it to make sure it is tender, not gritty), stir in the chorizo, onion, peppers and prawns, and season with salt and pepper. Divide between warmed bowls, scatter with the parsley and serve with a lemon wedge on the side.

PER SERVING

CALORIES	FAT	SAT FAT	CARBS	SUGARS	FIBRE	PROTEIN	SALT
505	11G	3.3G	68G	7.6G	4.2G	31G	2.6G

WORCESTERSHIRE ROAST BEEF

SERVES 6
PREP TIME 10 minutes, plus marinating and resting time
COOK TIME 42–52 minutes

4 tablespoons Worcestershire sauce

3 tablespoons dark soy sauce

juice of 1 lemon

5 garlic cloves, crushed

1 teaspoon cracked black pepper

beef roasting joint, about 950g (2lb 2oz) total weight, such as topside, silverside or top rump

The air fryer is perfect for getting an all-over sear on a joint of beef, and marinating it first will add delicious flavour as well as helping the meat to stay moist. My family loves this with Oxo Roast Potatoes or Mini Rosemary Roast Potatoes (see pages **142** and **145**) and everyone's favourite fresh vegetables. If you also want to cook your potatoes in the air fryer for the same meal, you can simply wrap the beef in foil and leave it to rest while they cook.

1 Make the marinade by mixing the Worcestershire sauce, soy sauce, lemon juice, crushed garlic and black pepper. I do this in a large zip-seal bag, then pop the beef joint in to marinate, but you can do it in a covered bowl or plastic food box if you prefer. Marinate for at least 2 hours, or overnight in the refrigerator if you have time, to really let the flavours infuse. I flip the beef joint over every now and again to ensure the marinade gets to every surface. Take the beef out of the refrigerator at least 30 minutes before you want to cook it.

2 Preheat 1 air fryer drawer to 200°C (400°F).

3 Place the beef in the drawer and cook for 12 minutes, then reduce the temperature to 180°C (350°F) and cook for 30 minutes (for medium-rare), turning the joint over halfway through the cooking time. If you want the beef well done, cook it for 40 minutes.

4 Remove the beef from the air fryer, cover with foil and let it rest for at least 30 minutes before carving so that the joint reabsorbs its juices and does not dry out.

PER SERVING

CALORIES	FAT	SAT FAT	CARBS	SUGARS	FIBRE	PROTEIN	SALT
307	6.5G	2.6G	5.9G	5.2G	0.5G	56G	2.6G

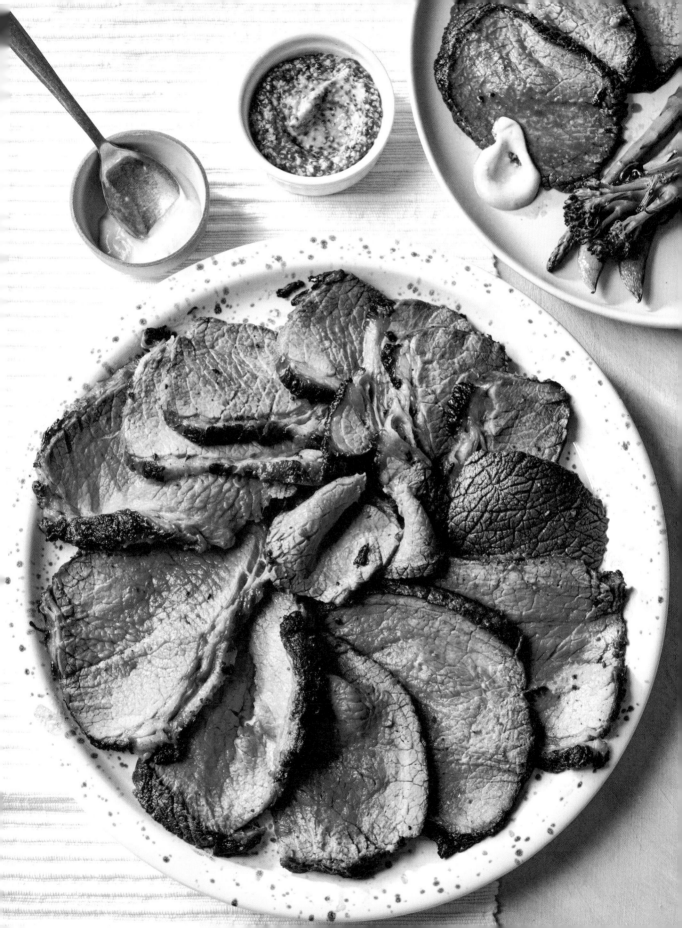

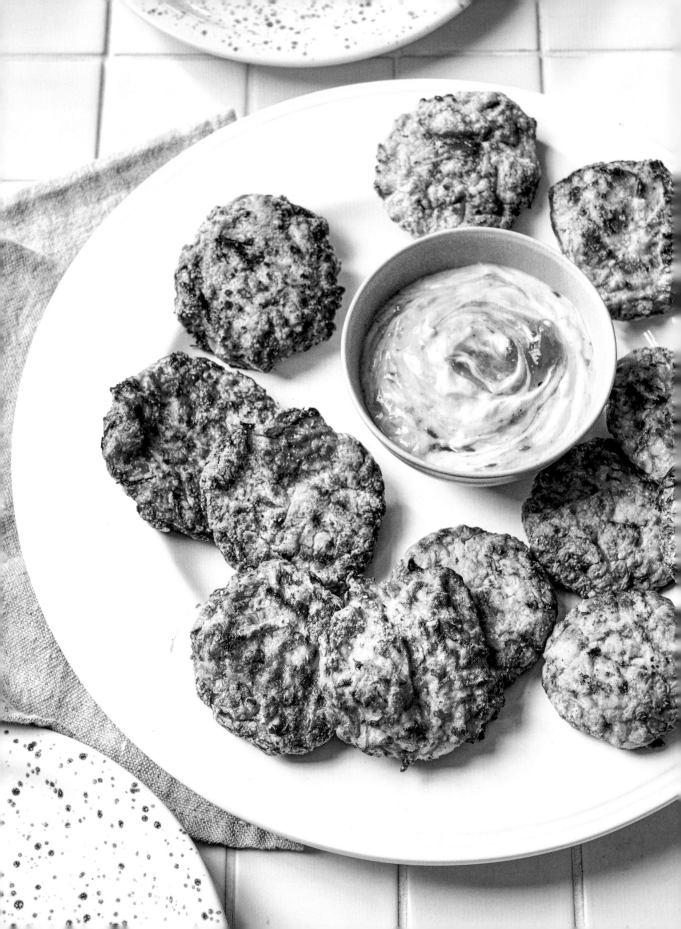

CURRIED CHICKEN RISSOLES

SERVES 4
PREP TIME 20 minutes
COOK TIME 20 minutes

500g (1lb 2oz) 5 per cent fat
   minced chicken
4 spring onions, finely sliced
2 garlic cloves, finely grated
5cm (2 inch) piece of fresh root
   ginger, peeled and finely grated
1 courgette, grated
1 carrot, grated
small handful of mint leaves,
   finely chopped
1 tablespoon mild or medium
   curry powder, as you prefer
1 egg, lightly beaten
4 tablespoons cornflour
spray oil
salt and pepper

FOR THE MANGO YOGURT DIP
4 tablespoons fat-free Greek
   yogurt
2 tablespoons mango chutney

Tasty chicken patties with a crisp exterior, these include grated carrot and courgette, so are a great way to get kids eating extra vegetables. These are delicious served with some warm flatbreads or naans, plus cucumber and carrot sticks on the side, or you could also serve them with basmati rice or couscous. Stir some peas through the rice with a little turmeric and cumin for extra flavour.

1 Put the chicken in a mixing bowl with the spring onions, garlic, ginger, courgette, carrot, mint, curry powder and egg. Season and stir everything together until all the ingredients are well combined.

2 Spread the cornflour on a small plate and have a dinner plate to hand.

3 Wet your hands before shaping the rissoles – this will help prevent the mixture from sticking to you. Using an ice-cream scoop, place a scoop of mixture in the palm of your hand. Shape it into a ball, then press down to create a round patty.

4 Dip both sides of each rissole into the cornflour, then place on the dinner plate. Repeat until you have 12 rissoles. Spray the top of the rissoles with oil, making sure you have good coverage so that they can crisp as they cook.

5 Preheat both air fryer drawers to 180°C (350°F). Spray the crisper plates with oil and carefully place 6 rissoles on each one with a little space between them. If they don't all fit, you might need to cook them in 2 batches.

6 Cook for 20 minutes, using silicone tongs to carefully flip the rissoles over halfway through to ensure even crispness.

7 Meanwhile, mix the yogurt, mango chutney and a pinch of salt in a small bowl. Serve the rissoles with the mango yogurt for dipping.

PER SERVING

CALORIES	FAT	SAT FAT	CARBS	SUGARS	FIBRE	PROTEIN	SALT
356	9.4G	2.4G	25G	9.9G	3G	41G	1.1G

HONEY BARBECUE HEDGEHOG CHICKEN

SERVES 4
PREP TIME 10 minutes
COOK TIME 20 minutes

4 skinless chicken breast fillets
2 tablespoons barbecue sauce
  (see page 96 for homemade)
1 tablespoon honey
1 teaspoon paprika
1 teaspoon garlic granules
½ teaspoon coarsely ground salt
spray oil

Super-quick to pull together, the chicken here is glazed with a flavoursome honey barbecue sauce. This will work with whatever sides you fancy, salad, fries, sweet potato, rice, couscous or roasted vegetables.

1   To 'hedgehog' the chicken, use a sharp knife to score each breast all the way across on the diagonal, cutting about three-quarters of the way through the flesh and spacing the cuts about 1cm (½ inch) apart. Then repeat, cutting diagonally across the breast in the opposite direction to create a cross-hatch pattern.

2   Preheat both air fryer drawers to 180°C (350°F).

3   In a small bowl, mix the barbecue sauce and honey. Use a teaspoon to smother the sauce over the cut side of the chicken, spreading it evenly over all 4 breasts and getting it down into the cuts. Sprinkle over the paprika, garlic granules and salt.

4   Place 2 chicken breasts in each air fryer drawer and spray the tops with oil. Cook for 20 minutes, then serve with your chosen accompaniments.

PER SERVING

CALORIES	FAT	SAT FAT	CARBS	SUGARS	FIBRE	PROTEIN	SALT
212	2.3G	0.5G	7.2G	6.6G	0	40G	1G

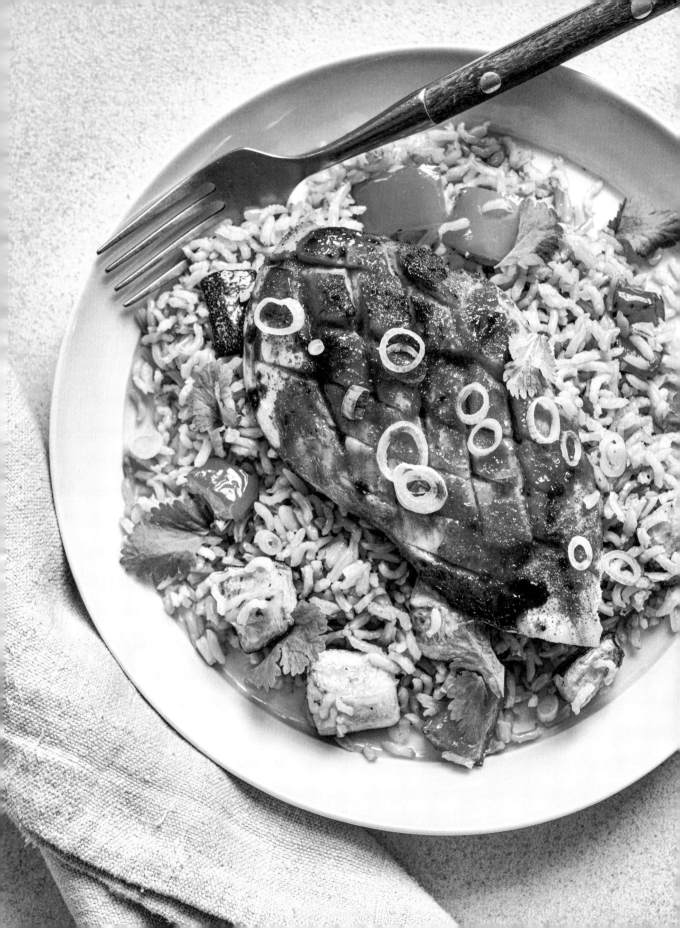

PERFECT STEAK

SERVES 4
PREP TIME 5 minutes
COOK TIME 8–12 minutes

4 ribeye or sirloin steaks (about
225g / 8oz each)
spray oil
salt and pepper

FOR THE SALSA VERDE
1 large garlic clove
3 canned anchovy fillets, patted
dry with kitchen paper and
roughly chopped
finely grated zest of 1 lemon
large handful of parsley
large handful of basil
small handful of mint leaves
1 tablespoon capers
1 teaspoon Dijon mustard
2 tablespoons red wine vinegar
1 teaspoon olive oil
1 ice cube

You really can cook a perfect steak in the air fryer because you can get
a great quick sear with the high temperature and the steak will cook
evenly on all sides. You can also cook 4 steaks all at once using both
drawers. I love steak with a fresh and zingy salsa verde. Serve with the
sides of your choice, a fresh salad or some homemade fries are perfect.

1   Remove the steak from the refrigerator at least 30 minutes before
    cooking.

2   Preheat both air fryer drawers to 200°C (400°F).

3   Spray each steak with oil on both sides and season with salt and pepper.
    Lay 2 steaks in each drawer by placing them at a diagonal angle, you
    should be able to fit them in easily, but don't overlap them. Cook for
    6 minutes, then use silicone tongs to flip them over and cook for an
    extra 2 minutes. This should give you a lovely medium-rare result.
    For medium, give them an extra 2 minutes, or for well done, another
    2 minutes. (Obviously steaks vary in thickness, so you may need to
    slightly adjust these cooking times to get the perfect result for you.)

4   Transfer the steaks to a warm plate and let them rest for a few minutes
    while you prepare the salsa verde.

5   Place all the salsa ingredients in a mini chopper or blender and purée
    until you have a smooth sauce. The ice will help to keep the herbs a
    bright, vivid green.

6   Serve the steak drizzled with salsa verde, or serve the sauce on the side
    if you prefer.

PER SERVING

CALORIES	FAT	SAT FAT	CARBS	SUGARS	FIBRE	PROTEIN	SALT
525	36G	15G	1.6G	1.4G	0.5G	49G	1.9G

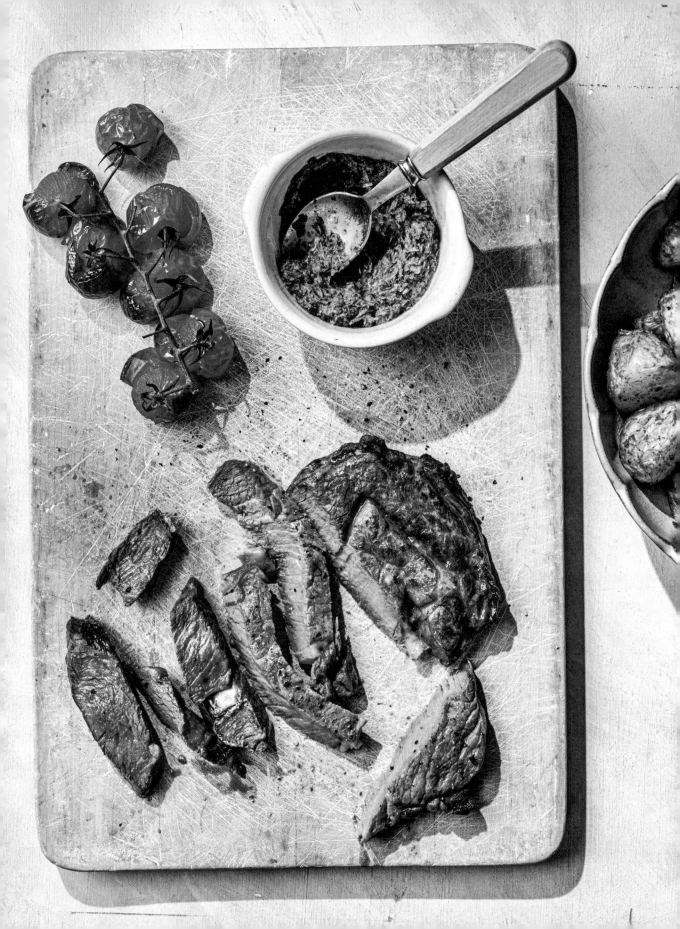

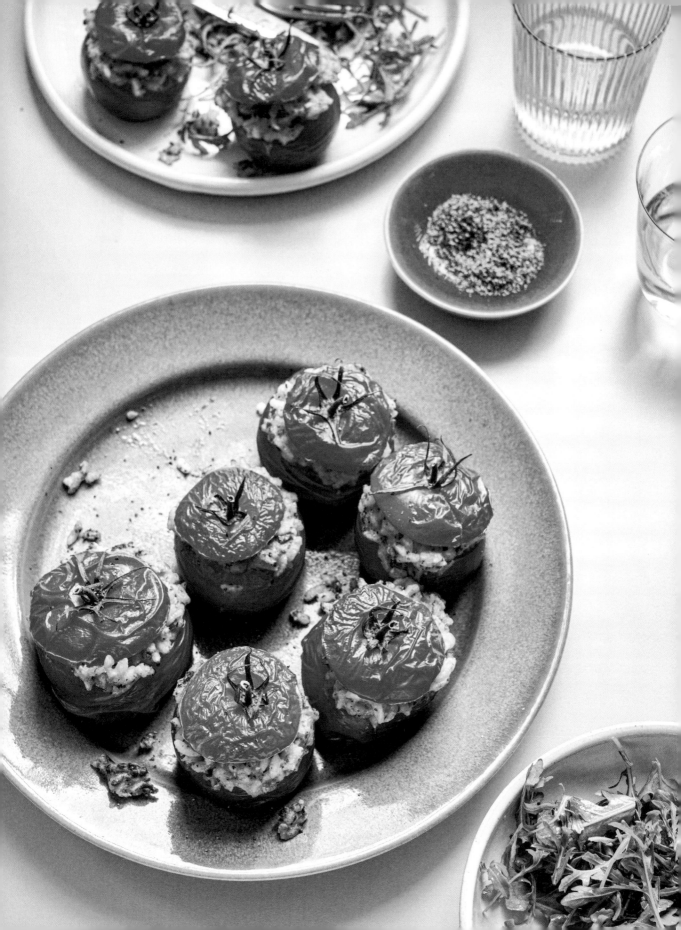

ROCKET PESTO STUFFED TOMATOES

SERVES 4
PREP TIME 20 minutes
COOK TIME 20 minutes

200g (7oz) risotto rice

8 vine tomatoes

handful of rocket, plus more to serve

2 garlic cloves, finely grated

50g (1¾oz) Parmesan-style vegetarian cheese, finely grated

20g (¾oz) sunflower seeds

2 tablespoons olive oil

salt and pepper

lemon wedges, to serve

A tasty twist on a family favourite, these tomatoes, filled with a mixture of risotto rice, rocket and Parmesan, are easy to prepare, and perfect for a comforting and simple meal. Enjoy with a rocket salad on the side, to underscore that flavour.

1   Bring a pot of salted water to the boil and cook the risotto rice for 10 minutes. Drain and set aside.

2   Slice the top off each of the tomatoes. Scoop the insides into a bowl. Add the rocket, garlic, Parmesan, sunflower seeds and olive oil. Whizz with a blender, but it doesn't have to be completely smooth. Mix this through the rice and season well with salt and pepper.

3   Preheat both air fryer drawers to 200°C (400°F).

4   Place 4 hollowed-out tomatoes in each drawer and cook for 3 minutes.

5   Scoop the rice mixture into the partially cooked tomatoes and place the tomato lids on top. If there is any extra rice mix, put this into a ramekin and cook alongside the tomatoes.

6   Reduce the temperature in both air fryer drawers to 190°C (375°F) and cook for 6 minutes.

7   Let the stuffed tomatoes sit for 10 minutes before eating. They may look a little watery at first, but all the juices will be absorbed by the rice as they sit. Serve with rocket, lemon wedges and grindings of black pepper.

PER SERVING

CALORIES	FAT	SAT FAT	CARBS	SUGARS	FIBRE	PROTEIN	SALT
330	13G	3.8G	42G	2.8G	2.1G	9.5G	0.33G

CHIPOTLE CHICKEN BURGERS WITH GARLIC-LIME SAUCE

SPECIAL CHOW MEIN

THAI-STYLE PRAWN & PINEAPPLE FRIED RICE

CHINESE-STYLE CHILLI BEEF

CHICKEN KATSU CURRY

CREAMY CASHEW CHICKEN CURRY

CRISPY HOISIN CHICKEN

SIZZLING KOREAN-STYLE PORK BALLS

CRISPY GOCHUJANG TOFU WITH CRUNCHY SALAD

CHEEKY PERI-PERI CHICKEN WITH CORN ON THE COB

CHEESY CHICKEN KYIVS

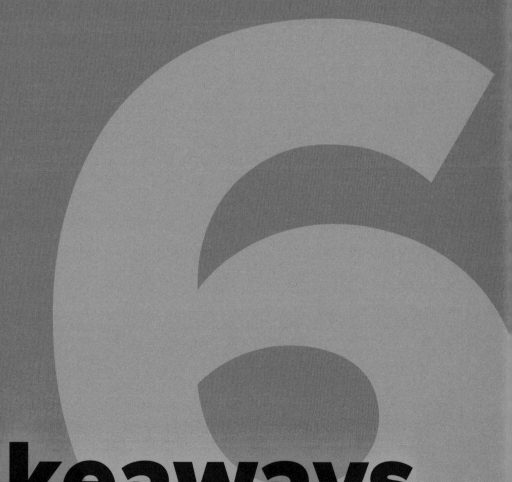

Fakeaways

CHIPOTLE CHICKEN BURGERS WITH GARLIC-LIME SAUCE

SERVES 4
PREP TIME 15 minutes
COOK TIME 12–14 minutes

2 skinless chicken breast fillets
40g (1½oz) puffed rice cereal
2 teaspoons chipotle paste
1 egg, lightly beaten
spray oil
4 brioche buns
salt and pepper

FOR THE BURGER SAUCE
200g (7oz) fat-free Greek yogurt
finely grated zest of 1 lime, plus
    1 tablespoon lime juice
1 teaspoon garlic powder
1 teaspoon onion granules
1 teaspoon honey

TO SERVE (OPTIONAL)
cheese slices
lettuce leaves
sliced tomato

Breakfast cereal used as a 'crumb' here provides a perfect crispy coating for chicken, and the combination of ingredients is a total winner. Chipotle chilli paste is widely available in supermarkets and lends a delicious smoky heat to this chicken burger, which is complemented with a fresh and zingy garlic-lime burger sauce. I've used brioche rolls as a treat, but you can choose a lower-calorie burger bun if you prefer.

1   Cut the chicken breasts in half to create 4 roughly equal pieces. Place 1 piece on a chopping board (I use a specific board for meat), cover with clingfilm or baking paper and bash with a rolling pin, or the base of a saucepan, to flatten it out to a uniform thickness of around 1cm (½ inch). Repeat with the other chicken pieces.

2   Put the rice cereal in a food processor with the chipotle paste and some salt and pepper, then whizz to form fine crumbs. Put the crumbs in a wide, shallow bowl (I use a pasta bowl) and use a separate bowl for the beaten egg. Dip each chicken piece into the egg, shake off any excess, then coat in the chipotle crumbs, making sure both sides are evenly coated.

3   Preheat both air fryer drawers to 200°C (400°F).

4   Spray the crisper plates in the air fryer with oil, then add the 4 chicken burgers to the air fryer drawers and spray them with oil, too. Cook for 10–12 minutes, turning halfway through, until the burgers are cooked through on the inside and crispy on the outside. The internal temperature of the thickest part of the burger shouldbe at least 75°C (167°F).

5   Meanwhile, make the burger sauce by mixing all the ingredients together in a small bowl.

6   Remove the chicken burgers from the air fryer. Slice open the brioche buns, place in the air fryer drawers and cook for 2 minutes to lightly toast them. Alternatively, you can do this under a grill, in a toaster or in a frying pan while the burgers are cooking.

7   Spread some burger sauce over the bottom half of each bun, add the burger, any other fillings, such as cheese slices, lettuce or tomato, then finish by adding the top of the bun.

PER SERVING

CALORIES	FAT	SAT FAT	CARBS	SUGARS	FIBRE	PROTEIN	SALT
364	6.6G	1.5G	41G	8.2G	1.6G	34G	0.92G

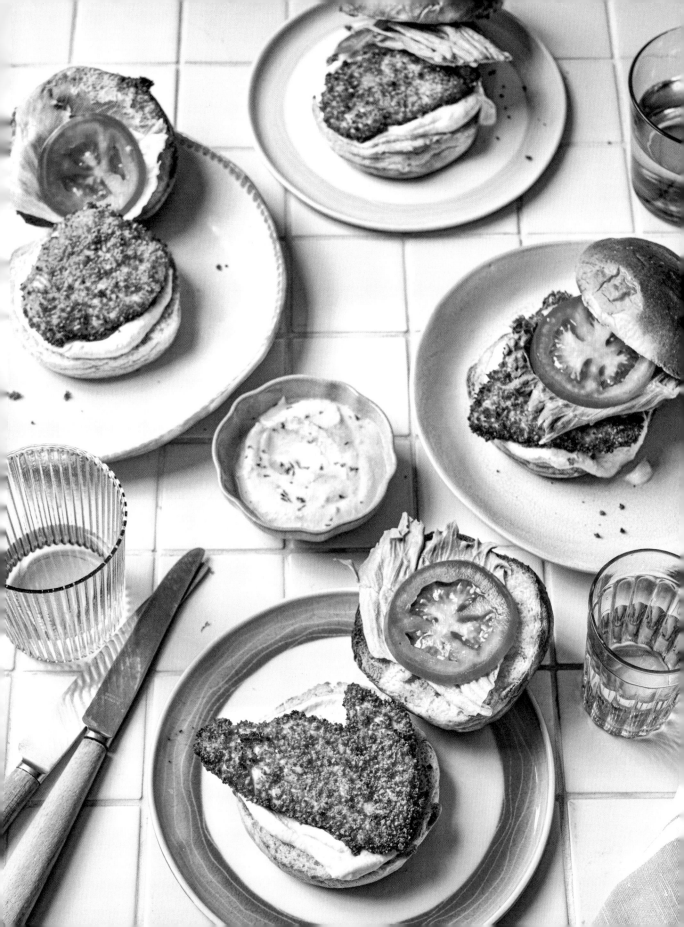

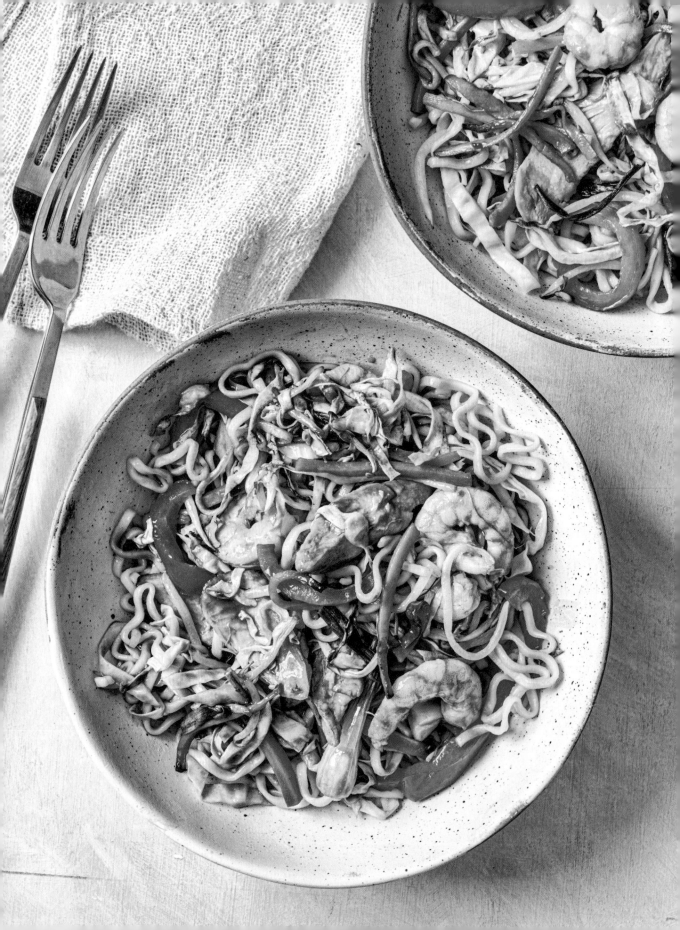

SPECIAL CHOW MEIN

SERVES 4
PREP TIME 15 minutes
COOK TIME 25 minutes

2 skinless chicken breast fillets

spray oil

bunch of spring onions, trimmed and sliced

2 carrots, cut into matchsticks

1 red pepper, deseeded and cut into matchsticks

1 teaspoon sesame oil

200g (7oz) dried medium egg noodles

150g (5½oz) sweetheart (pointed/ Hispi) cabbage, finely shredded

150g (5½oz) cold-water prawns, defrosted

100g (3½oz) beansprouts

FOR THE SAUCE

1 tablespoon cornflour

3 tablespoons cold water

3 tablespoons oyster sauce

3 tablespoons dark soy sauce

1 tablespoon apple cider vinegar

1 teaspoon sesame oil

A thoroughly tasty combination of chicken, prawns and noodles with mixed vegetables in a dark and savoury sauce. Make sure you have all the veg prepped before you start, to help this go smoothly.

1 Preheat 1 air fryer drawer to 180°C (350°F). Spray the chicken breasts with oil and cook them for 18–20 minutes, turning halfway through.

2 In a small bowl, make up the sauce: stir the cornflour into the cold water to ensure it doesn't clump, then add it to the other sauce ingredients and mix well.

3 Once the chicken has been cooking for 10 minutes, remove the crisper plate from the second drawer and preheat that drawer to 200°C (400°F). Put the spring onions, carrots and pepper in the drawer, drizzle with the sesame oil and cook for 10 minutes, stirring every few minutes.

4 Meanwhile, cook the noodles on the hob according to the packet instructions. Be sure not to overcook them as you don't want them sticking together. Drain the noodles, then spray them with a few sprays of oil, tossing as you go, to prevent them from clumping.

5 Once the chicken breasts are cooked through (they should have reached an internal temperature of 75°C / 167°F), slice them thinly.

6 Remove the crisper plate from the drawer used for the chicken (careful as it will be hot), then divide the spring onion mixture equally between the 2 drawers and set the temperature of each to 200°C (400°F). Add the cabbage, prawns and beansprouts to the drawers, splitting them equally, spray with oil and cook for 2 minutes.

7 Divide the noodles, chicken and sauce evenly between the drawers, give everything a good toss with silicone tongs and cook for 3 minutes, tossing again halfway through. Once everything is hot (give it a couple more minutes if the noodles aren't fully reheated), serve straight away.

PER SERVING

CALORIES	FAT	SAT FAT	CARBS	SUGARS	FIBRE	PROTEIN	SALT
400	6.5G	1.1G	48G	11G	6.8G	34G	3.4G

THAI-STYLE PRAWN & PINEAPPLE FRIED RICE

SERVES 4
PREP TIME 15 minutes
COOK TIME 20 minutes

425g (15oz) can of pineapple chunks, drained, each chunk cut into 4

spray oil

1 onion, finely chopped

1 red pepper, deseeded and finely chopped

1 teaspoon sesame oil

1 red birds eye chilli, finely chopped

2 garlic cloves, crushed

200g (7oz) raw king prawns, patted dry with kitchen paper

500g (1lb 2oz) cooked, cold jasmine rice (200g / 7oz raw)

180g (6oz) mangetout or sugar snap peas

150g (5½oz) frozen petits pois

2 tablespoons dark soy sauce

1 tablespoon fish sauce

1 teaspoon demerara sugar

2 eggs, lightly beaten

4 spring onions, sliced

2 teaspoons sesame seeds

The air fryer gives a lovely level of caramelization and char to pineapple chunks in this flavoursome stir-fry. If you prefer, you can use fresh pineapple, but I usually go for canned for convenience.

1 Remove the crisper plate from 1 of the air fryer drawers and preheat both drawers to 200°C (400°F).

2 Place the pineapple chunks in an even layer in the drawer with the crisper plate and spray with oil. Cook for 20 minutes, stirring halfway through.

3 Put the onion, pepper and sesame oil into the other drawer, stir and cook for 5 minutes. Add the chilli and garlic, stir, then lay the prawns on top. Spray them with some oil and cook for 5 minutes.

4 Add the cooked cold rice, mangetout, petits pois, soy sauce, fish sauce and demerara sugar in with the prawn mixture, stir well, then push it all towards one end of the drawer to create a little space for the beaten eggs: these need to be in contact with the bottom of the drawer. Cook for 5 minutes, check the egg is mostly cooked, then stir it into the rest of the ingredients, breaking it up. If there is still any raw egg, cook for another couple of minutes.

5 Stir the pineapple through the rice, then divide between 4 warmed bowls, scattering with spring onions and sesame seeds.

PER SERVING

CALORIES	FAT	SAT FAT	CARBS	SUGARS	FIBRE	PROTEIN	SALT
388	6.5G	1.4G	58G	19G	6.7G	21G	2.3G

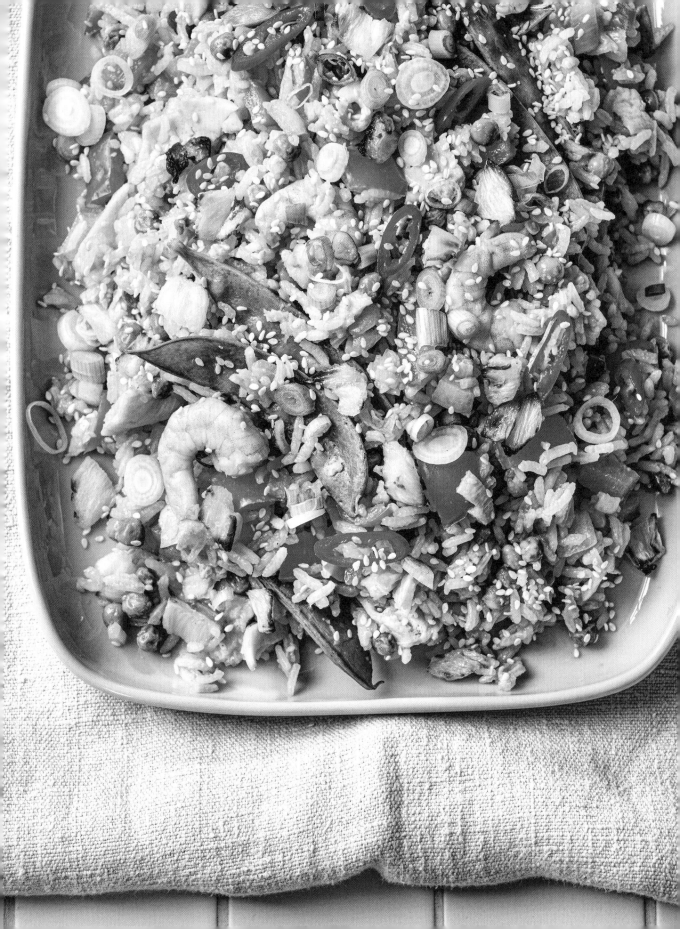

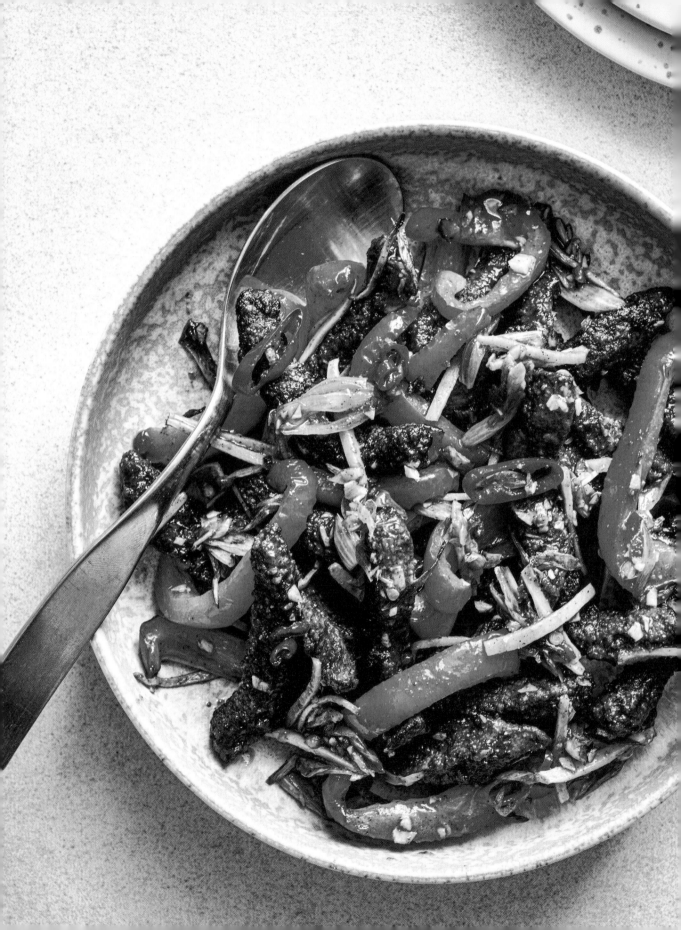

CHINESE-STYLE CHILLI BEEF

SERVES 4
PREP TIME 10 minutes
COOK TIME 23 minutes

400g (14oz) thin cut steak, larger pieces of fat discarded, sliced into strips

1½ tablespoons cornflour

2 teaspoons Chinese 5 spice

spray oil

1 red chilli, finely sliced

1 red pepper, deseeded and finely sliced

3cm piece of fresh root ginger, peeled and cut into thin matchsticks

4 spring onions, finely sliced

3 tablespoons rice vinegar

1 teaspoon sesame oil

2 garlic cloves, crushed

1 tablespoon sweet chilli sauce

1 tablespoon light soy sauce

1 tablespoon tomato ketchup

This is a quick and delicious meal, perfect for air frying. The thinly sliced steak is seasoned and cooked to crispy perfection, before being paired with vegetables and a tangy sauce.

1   Place the beef strips in a bowl and stir in the cornflour and Chinese 5 spice.

2   Preheat both air fryer drawers to 200°C (400°F). Spray the crisper plates with oil, then add the beef strips, allowing a little space between each strip so it has a chance to crisp up. Spray the beef with oil, then cook for 6 minutes. Turn the beef strips over and cook for another 4 minutes.

3   Remove the beef from the air fryer and set aside in a warm bowl covered with foil.

4   Remove the crisper plate from 1 drawer and add the chilli, red pepper, ginger and spring onions, 1 tablespoon of the rice vinegar and the sesame oil. Stir well and air fry for 10 minutes, stirring a couple of times during cooking and adding the garlic for the last 2 minutes.

5   In a small bowl, mix together the remaining 2 tablespoons of rice vinegar, the sweet chilli sauce, soy sauce and tomato ketchup.

6   Once the vegetables have cooked for 10 minutes, return the beef to the air fryer, stir through the sauce and heat for 3 minutes before serving, over basmati rice, if you like.

PER SERVING

CALORIES	FAT	SAT FAT	CARBS	SUGARS	FIBRE	PROTEIN	SALT
218	6.3G	2.2G	13G	7.3G	1.7G	25G	1G

CHICKEN KATSU CURRY

SERVES 4
PREP TIME 20 minutes
COOK TIME 45 minutes

4 skinless chicken breast fillets
  (about 150g / 5½oz each)
50g (1¾oz) cornflakes, finely
  crushed
1 egg, lightly beaten
salt and pepper

FOR THE CURRY SAUCE
spray oil
2 onions, finely chopped
5 garlic cloves, roughly chopped
1 tablespoon plain flour
4 teaspoons curry powder
600ml (20fl oz) hot chicken stock
2 carrots, finely sliced
2 teaspoons honey
4 teaspoons light soy sauce
1 teaspoon garam masala

This has always been one of the most popular recipes on my blog, and was developed to replicate my favourite restaurant katsu curry. The sauce is made on the hob, while cornflake-coated chicken crisps to perfection in the air fryer. I like to serve this with basmati rice and edamame beans.

1   Start by making the curry sauce. Heat some spray oil in a medium nonstick saucepan on the hob, add the onions and cook until softened. Stir in the garlic and stir-fry for another minute. Add the flour and curry powder and cook, stirring, for 1 minute. Gradually pour in the hot stock, then add the carrots to the pan, along with the honey and soy sauce. Slowly bring to the boil.

2   Reduce the heat and simmer for 20 minutes, or until the sauce thickens a little but is still of pouring consistency. Stir in the garam masala. Whizz the sauce with a stick blender until it is completely smooth. Leave to simmer on a very low heat while you cook the chicken, stirring occasionally.

3   Lay some baking paper or clingfilm over the chicken breasts one at a time, then bash with a rolling pin or the base of a saucepan to flatten them to about 1cm (½ inch) thick.

4   Put the crushed cornflakes into a wide shallow bowl and the egg in another. Dip each chicken breast in the egg, shaking off the excess, then dip in the cornflake crumbs, making sure it's thoroughly coated. Place on a plate while you crumb the remaining chicken. Season with salt and pepper, then spray with some oil.

5   Preheat both air fryer drawers to 180°C (350°F). Spray the crisper plates with oil, then place 2 crumbed chicken breasts in each drawer. Cook for 10 minutes, then use silicone tongs to carefully turn each piece of chicken over and cook for another 6 minutes. The chicken should be golden and crisp on the outside and cooked through in the middle (you can check that it's done with a food thermometer: the internal temperature should be at least 75°C / 167°F).

6   When you're ready to serve, use a sharp knife to slice the chicken breasts into 1cm (½ inch) slices and arrange neatly on plates. Pour the sauce over to serve, with some edamame beans and basmati rice on the side.

PER SERVING

CALORIES	FAT	SAT FAT	CARBS	SUGARS	FIBRE	PROTEIN	SALT
350	4.2G	1.1G	29G	13G	5.7G	46G	2.3G

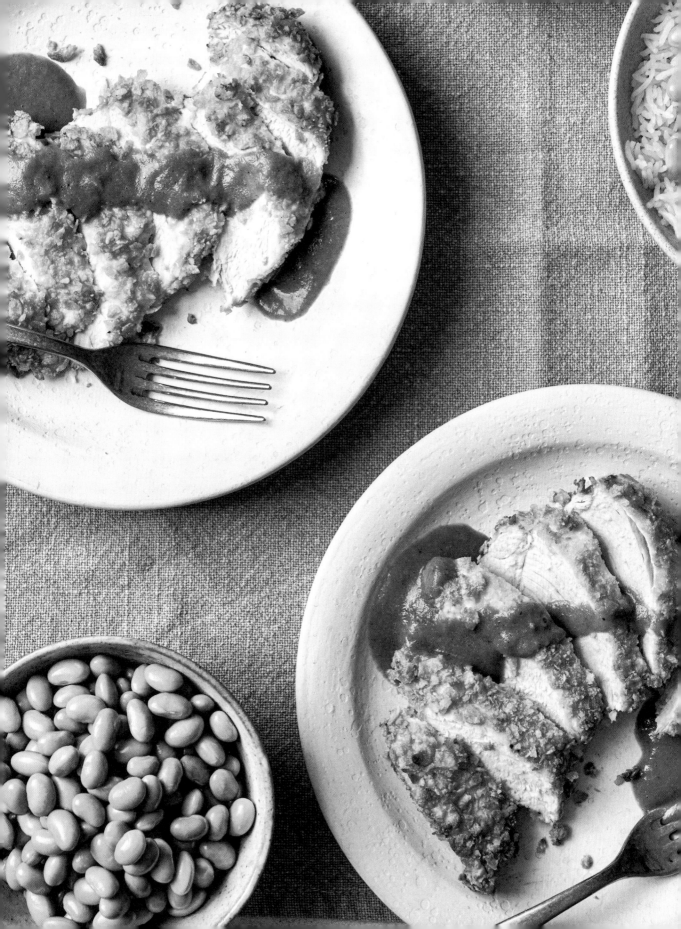

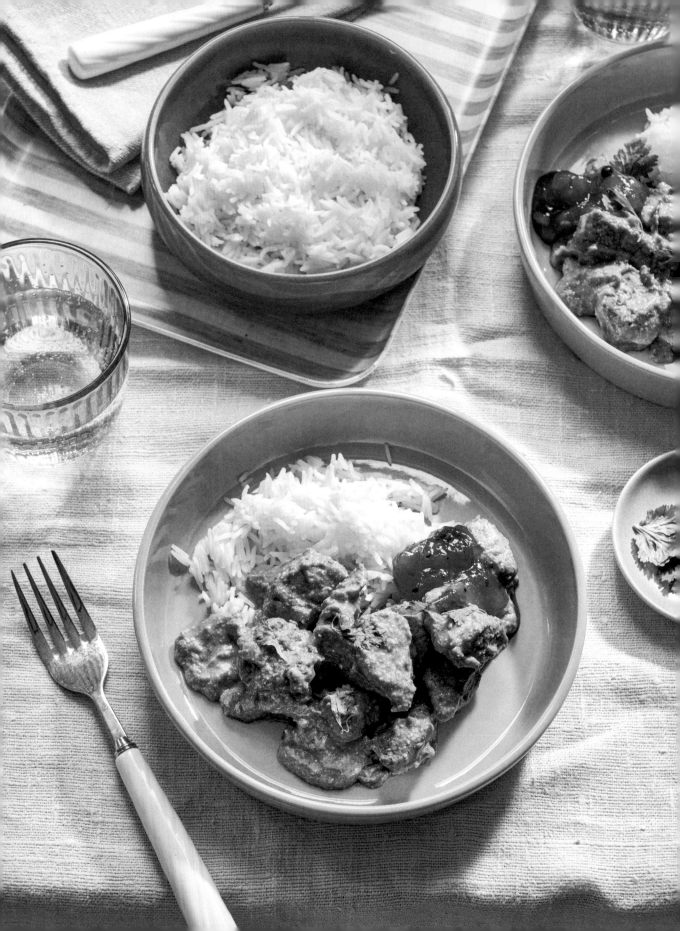

CREAMY CASHEW CHICKEN CURRY

SERVES 4
PREP TIME 15 minutes
COOK TIME 30 minutes

4 skinless chicken breast fillets, chopped
1 large onion, finely chopped
2 teaspoons olive oil
75g (2¾oz) whole cashew nuts
300ml (10fl oz) cold water
400g (14oz) can of chopped tomatoes
2 garlic cloves, crushed
5cm (2 inch) piece of fresh root ginger, peeled and finely grated
85g (3oz) fat-free Greek yogurt
1 tablespoon cornflour
juice of 1 lime
coriander leaves, to serve

FOR THE SPICE MIX
1 teaspoon paprika
1 teaspoon garam masala
1 teaspoon ground cumin
1 teaspoon coarsely ground salt
½ teaspoon ground coriander
½ teaspoon ground turmeric
¼ teaspoon cayenne pepper

Puréed cashew nuts form the creamy base of this curry. With a mild level of heat, it will be a winner with the whole family. Serve with fluffy basmati rice.

1 Make the spice mix by combining all the ingredients for it in a bowl.

2 In a mixing bowl, stir together the chicken, onion, olive oil and half the spice mix. Leave that to marinate while you prepare the nuts.

3 Remove the crisper plates and preheat 1 of the drawers to 200°C (400°F). Tip the cashews into the drawer and cook for 5 minutes. They should be lightly toasted, with just a hint of golden brown. Once toasted, tip them into a food processor or blender.

4 Preheat the second air fryer drawer to 200°C (400°F). Divide the spiced chicken and onion mixture between the 2 drawers, spreading it in an even layer. Cook for 12 minutes, stirring halfway through.

5 Meanwhile, add the measured cold water to the food processor or blender and whizz until the cashews are as smooth as you can get them. Now pour in the chopped tomatoes and blend again until you have a smooth sauce.

6 Once the chicken has cooked for 12 minutes, divide the garlic, ginger and the rest of the spice mix between the 2 drawers, stir and cook for 2 minutes.

7 In a small bowl, stir the yogurt and cornflour until combined without any lumps.

8 Pour half the cashew sauce and yogurt mixture into each air fryer drawer, stir, then reduce the temperature to 180°C (350°F) and cook for 10 minutes, stirring halfway. The sauce should now be thick and creamy, and the chicken fully cooked. If you think the sauce needs to thicken up a little more, air fry for another 5 minutes.

9 Finally, stir the lime juice through the curry (dividing it between the 2 drawers) and serve, scattered with coriander.

PER SERVING

CALORIES	FAT	SAT FAT	CARBS	SUGARS	FIBRE	PROTEIN	SALT
375	13G	2.6G	16G	9.4G	3.9G	44G	1.5G

CRISPY HOISIN CHICKEN

SERVES 4
PREP TIME 20 minutes
COOK TIME 24 minutes

1 egg white

1 tablespoon cornflour

1½ teaspoons sesame oil

6–8 skinless chicken thigh fillets (total weight about 700g / 1lb 9oz), excess fat trimmed away, cut into bite-sized pieces

4 garlic cloves, crushed

5cm (2 inch) piece of fresh root ginger, peeled and finely grated

4 spring onions, finely sliced

2 tablespoons hoisin sauce

1 tablespoon Chinese rice wine

1 tablespoon light soy sauce

1 tablespoon honey

Crispy little bites of chicken in a flavoursome hoisin-based sauce makes a delicious, family-friendly fakeaway.

1   In a large bowl, beat together the egg white, cornflour and ½ teaspoon of the sesame oil until smooth. Stir in the chicken and leave to marinate for 15 minutes.

2   Preheat both air fryer drawers to 200°C (400°F).

3   Divide the chicken between the 2 drawers allowing a little space between each piece rather than being clumped together. Cook for 15 minutes.

4   Now transfer all the chicken into 1 drawer, mix, then cook for another 5 minutes.

5   In a small bowl, combine the garlic, ginger and spring onions with the remaining teaspoon of sesame oil. Carefully remove the crisper plate from the empty drawer (careful as it will be hot), put in the garlic mixture and cook for 2 minutes.

6   Mix the hoisin sauce, rice wine, soy sauce and honey in another small bowl. Once the garlic mix has cooked for 2 minutes, stir in the sauce and cook for 1 minute.

7   Now transfer the crispy chicken into the drawer with the sauce and mix thoroughly. Cook for 1 more minute before serving.

PER SERVING

CALORIES	FAT	SAT FAT	CARBS	SUGARS	FIBRE	PROTEIN	SALT
329	15G	4G	13G	7.9G	0.6G	36	1.3G

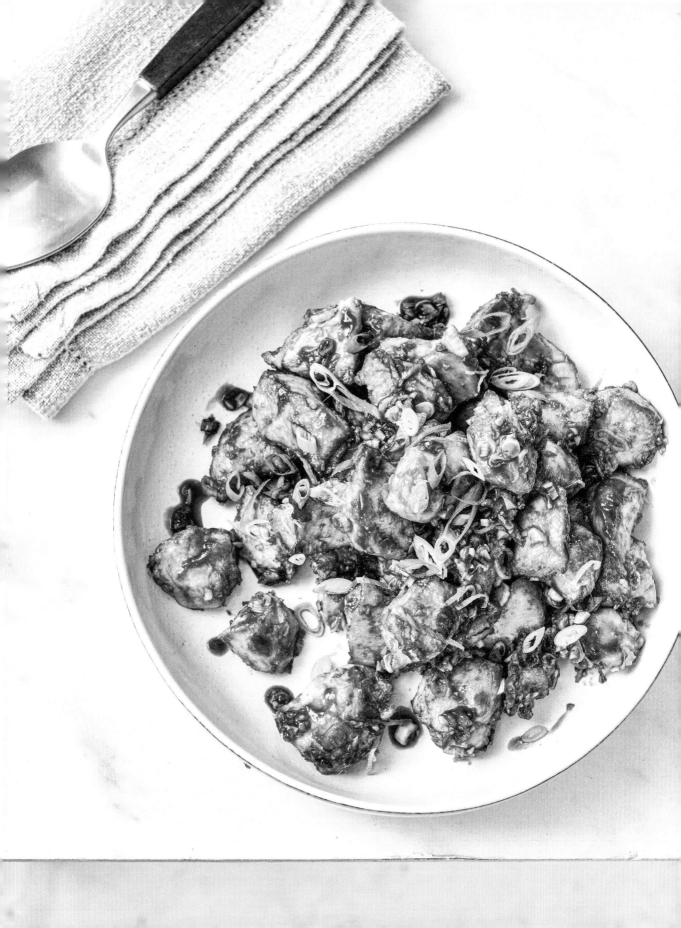

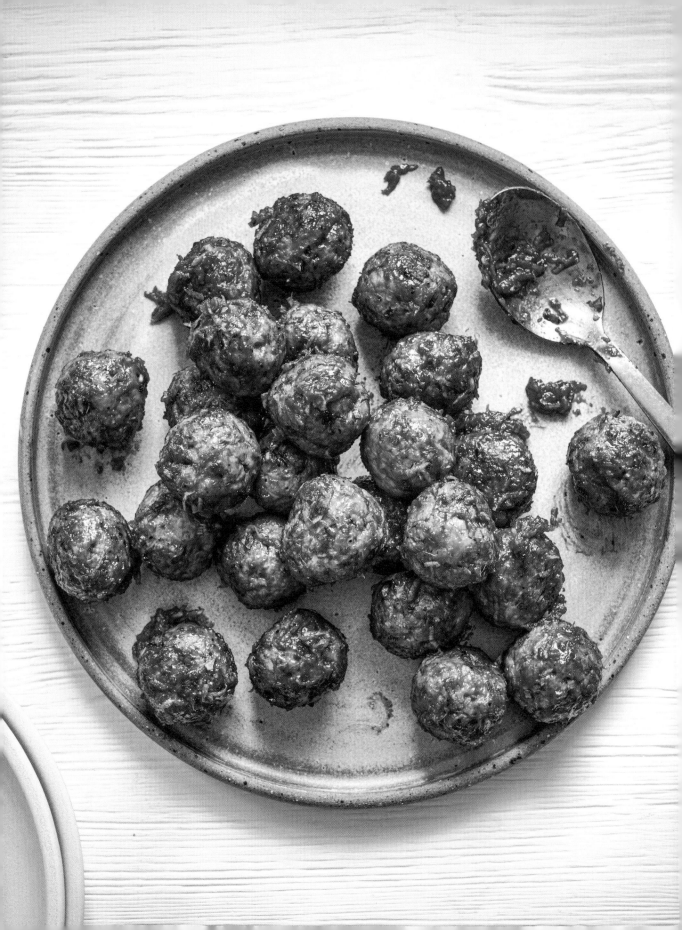

SIZZLING KOREAN-STYLE PORK BALLS

SERVES 4
PREP TIME 20 minutes
COOK TIME 17 minutes

500g (1lb 2oz) lean minced pork
   (5 per cent fat or less)
4 spring onions, trimmed and
   finely chopped
1 carrot, grated
2 garlic cloves, crushed
2cm (¾ inch) piece of fresh root
   ginger, peeled and finely grated
25g (1oz) panko breadcrumbs
1 egg, lightly beaten
salt and pepper
spray oil

FOR THE SAUCE
2 garlic cloves, crushed
2cm (¾ inch) piece of fresh root
   ginger, peeled and finely grated
1 tablespoon honey
1 tablespoon dark brown sugar
1 tablespoon rice wine
1 tablespoon gochujang paste
1 tablespoon apple cider vinegar
1 teaspoon sesame oil

Spicy, sweet and savoury, these tasty meatballs have it all. They are lovely served with basmati rice and Tenderstem broccoli.

1   Place the pork in a mixing bowl with the spring onions, carrot, garlic, ginger, panko, egg and some salt and pepper and mix thoroughly. Shape into 20–22 balls around 2.5cm (1 inch) in diameter.

2   Preheat both air fryer drawers to 180°C (350°F), divide the meatballs equally between them, spray with oil and air fry for 10 minutes.

3   Meanwhile, mix all the sauce ingredients in a small bowl.

4   Once the meatballs have cooked for 10 minutes, tip them all into the same drawer, then remove the crisper plate from the empty drawer (carefully, as it will be hot).

5   Put the sauce into the empty air fryer drawer and cook for 2 minutes.

6   Tip the sauce into the drawer with the meatballs and stir gently being careful not to break the meatballs apart as you do so, but ensure they are all covered with sauce. Now cook for a final 5 minutes, giving them a stir halfway through.

PER SERVING

CALORIES	FAT	SAT FAT	CARBS	SUGARS	FIBRE	PROTEIN	SALT
288	6.6G	1.9G	18G	13G	2.4G	37G	0.72G

CRISPY GOCHUJANG TOFU WITH CRUNCHY SALAD

SERVES 4
PREP TIME 15 minutes
COOK TIME 12 minutes

280g (10oz) extra-firm tofu

1 tablespoon gochujang paste

1 tablespoon soy sauce

2 teaspoons sesame oil

1 teaspoon garlic powder or granules

1 teaspoon onion powder or granules

2 tablespoons cornflour

1 teaspoon sesame seeds

lime wedges, to serve

FOR THE SAUCE

2 tablespoons gochujang paste

1 tablespoon honey

1½ tablespoons rice wine vinegar

1 garlic clove, finely grated

1 teaspoon sesame oil

FOR THE SALAD

2 Baby Gem lettuces, sliced

½ cucumber, halved lengthways, then sliced

2 spring onions, finely sliced

240g (8½oz) packet of radishes, very thinly sliced

1 carrot, grated

handful of coriander, chopped, plus extra to garnish

This crispy tofu is highly addictive, and the crunchy salad is the perfect foil to its sweet spice. There are so many flavours going on here that plain rice or noodles will complete the meal.

1 Drain the tofu and slice into roughly 2–3cm (1 inch) cubes. Mix the gochujang paste in a bowl with the soy sauce, sesame oil, garlic powder and onion powder to form a paste. Stir in the tofu until completely coated. Add the cornflour and toss again until each piece is covered.

2 Preheat both air fryer drawers to 180°C (350°F).

3 Carefully line both hot drawers with nonstick baking paper, then distribute the tofu pieces between them. Cook for 10–12 minutes until crispy.

4 Mix the ingredients for the sauce in a bowl.

5 Combine all the salad ingredients in a large bowl.

6 Serve the tofu drizzled with the sauce and sprinkled with the sesame seeds and extra coriander. Serve the salad alongside and give a good squeeze of lime over everything.

PER SERVING

CALORIES	FAT	SAT FAT	CARBS	SUGARS	FIBRE	PROTEIN	SALT
236	9.9G	1.8G	22G	12G	4.1G	12G	1.5G

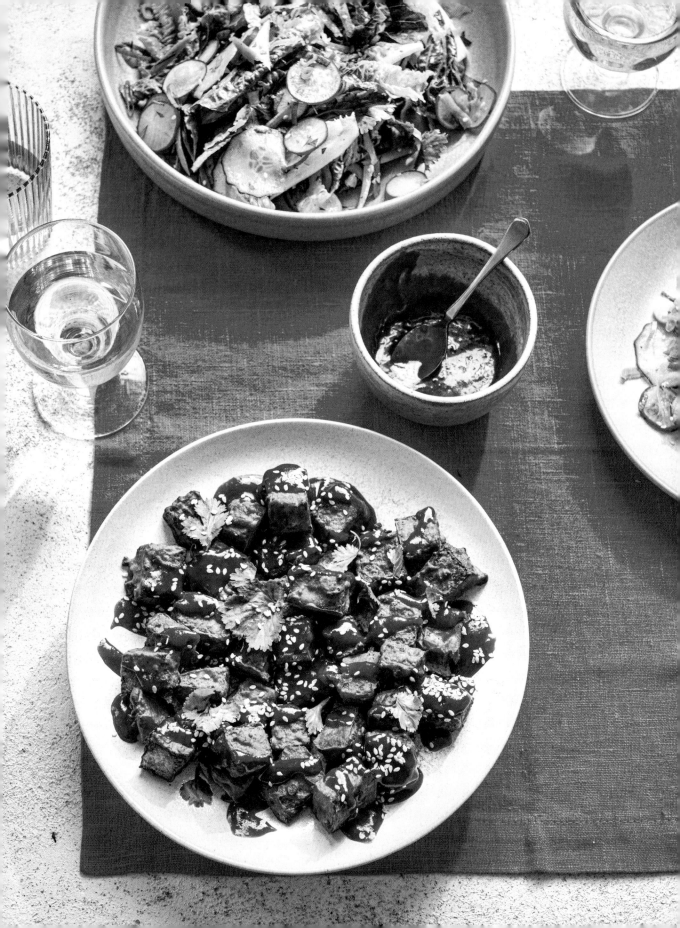

CHEEKY PERI-PERI CHICKEN WITH CORN ON THE COB

SERVES 4
PREP TIME 10 minutes
COOK TIME 30 minutes

---

2 peppers, deseeded and cut into quarters

spray oil

4 sweetcorn cobs

4 skinless chicken breast fillets, each cut lengthways into 4 pieces to form mini fillets

FOR THE PERI-PERI SPICE MIX

1 teaspoon paprika

1 teaspoon onion granules

1 teaspoon garlic powder or granules

1 teaspoon sugar (optional)

1 teaspoon ground coriander

½ teaspoon coarsely ground salt

½ teaspoon cracked black pepper

½ teaspoon dried parsley

½ teaspoon dried oregano

½ teaspoon crushed chilli flakes (double this if you like it spicier)

½ teaspoon ground cumin

¼ teaspoon cayenne pepper

This has always been a real favourite on The Slimming Foodie blog, and it's perfect for the air fryer as you get those lovely charred edges on the chicken. Serve this with a salad, or with fries or spicy rice if you prefer.

1 Preheat 1 air fryer drawer to 200°C (400°F) and the other to 190°C (375°F). Add the peppers, skin side down, to the hotter drawer, spray with oil and cook for 18 minutes. Put the corn cobs in the other drawer, spray with oil and cook for 12–14 minutes.

2 Combine all the ingredients for the spice mix in a large bowl and toss through the chicken pieces, making sure they are all evenly coated. Spray with oil, toss again and repeat a couple of times, so the chicken is all lightly covered in oil.

3 Once the peppers and sweetcorn are cooked, remove them from the drawers and set aside. Set both drawers to 200°C (400°F).

4 Place the chicken pieces in the air fryer drawers, allowing a little space between each. Cook for 12 minutes.

5 Remove the chicken from the drawers (I place it in a warmed bowl and cover with foil), pop the vegetables back in and reheat them for 2 minutes. Serve with the chicken.

PER SERVING

CALORIES	FAT	SAT FAT	CARBS	SUGARS	FIBRE	PROTEIN	SALT
274	4.3G	0.8G	13G	5.8G	4.7G	44G	0.8G

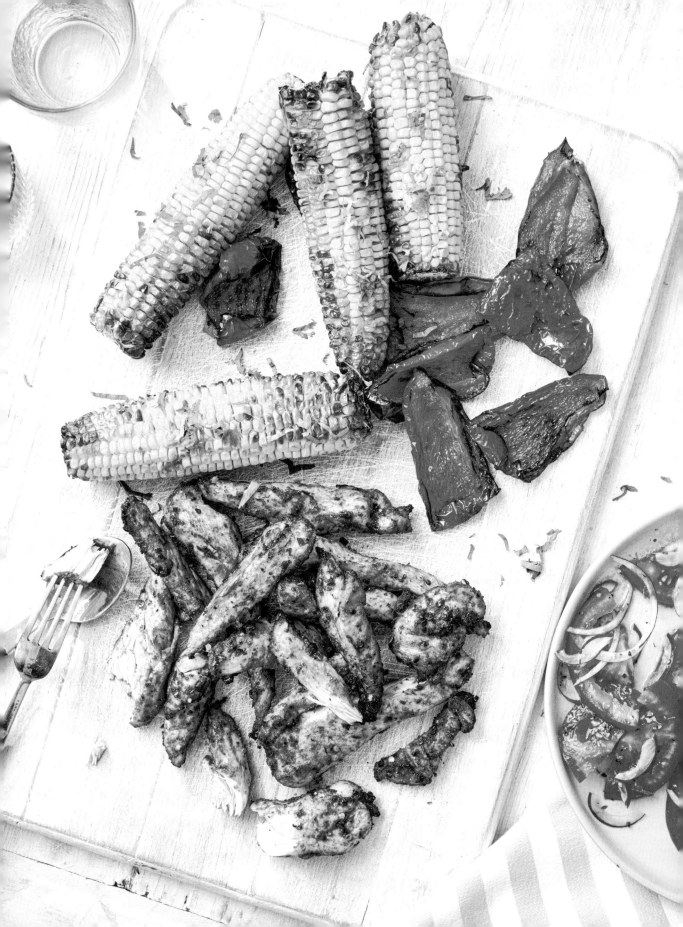

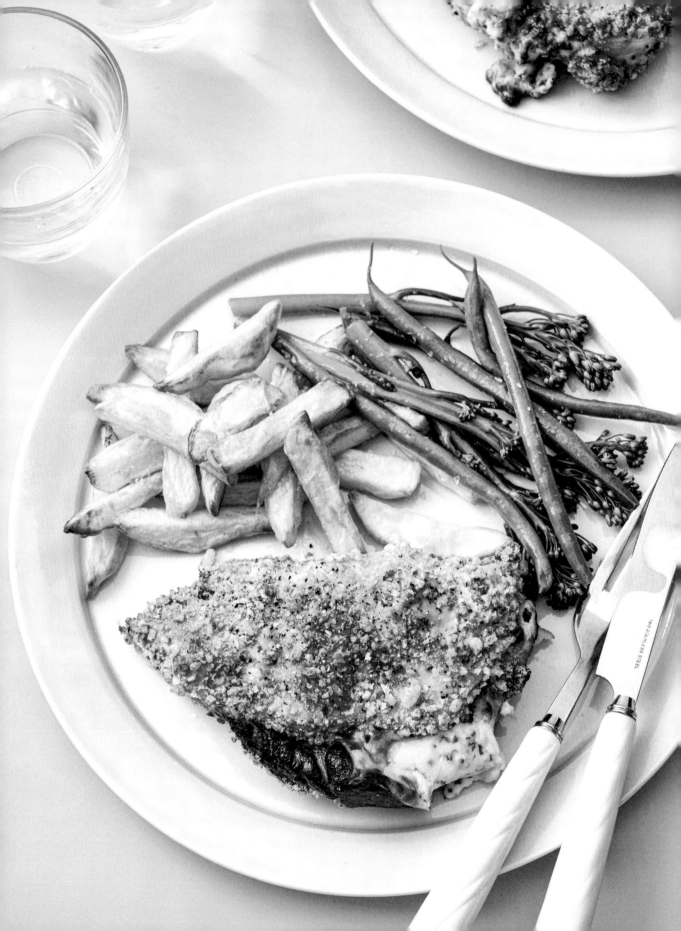

CHEESY CHICKEN KYIVS

SERVES 4
PREP TIME 15 minutes
COOK TIME 27 minutes

4 garlic cloves, crushed

spray oil

12 cheese triangles (I use Dairylea)

small handful of parsley leaves, finely chopped

60g (2¼oz) puffed rice cereal

1 egg, lightly beaten

4 skinless chicken breast fillets

salt and pepper

Chicken breasts stuffed with garlic and herb cheese are an indulgent-tasting treat that everyone will love. A light, crispy coating cooks perfectly in an air fryer, and any shop-bought kyiv pales in comparison. I specifically use cheese triangles here because they have the perfect consistency to become nice and melty without dribbling out of the chicken, so you don't lose all your filling while cooking these. My family like them with chips and peas!

1   Preheat 1 air fryer drawer to 200°C (400°F). Place the crushed garlic in a ramekin, spray it with a little bit of oil and air fry it for 2 minutes.

2   In a small bowl, use a fork to mash and mix the cheese triangles, cooked garlic and parsley.

3   Whizz the puffed rice cereal in a food processor to finely crush it, then pour it into a bowl. Put the egg into another bowl.

4   Slice the chicken horizontally through the middle with a sharp knife leaving it 'hinged' on one side. Spoon in the cheesy garlic mix, dividing it equally between the 4 breasts and gently pressing the chicken back down around it. (It doesn't matter if some filling is exposed.)

5   Dip the chicken breasts into the beaten egg, then roll through the crushed rice cereal to fully coat. Lay these on a plate as you go. Once they are all coated, season with salt and pepper and spray with oil.

6   Preheat both air fryer drawers to 180°C (350°F) and carefully place 2 kyiv in each drawer. Cook for 22–25 minutes, until golden and crisp on the outside and cooked through in the middle (you can check that it's done with a food thermometer: the internal temperature should be at least 75°C / 167°F).

PER SERVING

CALORIES	FAT	SAT FAT	CARBS	SUGARS	FIBRE	PROTEIN	SALT
351	9.9G	4.9G	14G	3.1G	0.9G	51G	0.2G

HONEY-SRIRACHA PEANUTS

OXO ROAST POTATOES

MINI ROSEMARY ROAST
POTATOES

EASY ROASTED RATATOUILLE

GOLDEN CHIPPIES

SOUTHWESTERN CORN
SALAD

FRIED EDAMAME

HOT HONEY

REFRIED BEANS

PERFECT CHIPS

SPICY PIZZA POPS

7

Sides, snacks & sauces

HONEY-SRIRACHA PEANUTS

SERVES 6 as a nibble
PREP TIME 5 minutes
COOK TIME 5 minutes

200g (7oz) roasted salted peanuts
1 teaspoon sriracha
1 teaspoon honey

I first whipped these up when I had forgotten to buy some snacks when friends were over for a drink. I took a boring bag of peanuts, added a couple of storecupboard flavourings and found the air fryer perfect for getting an all-over spicy honey glaze on to those nuts: they went down a storm, and now we often make them. This is a cost-effective alternative to buying fancy packs of crisps or nuts, and they can even be served warm as a real crowd pleaser.

1   Remove the crisper plate from 1 air fryer drawer and preheat that drawer to 200°C (400°F). Add the peanuts and cook for 2 minutes.

2   Shake the drawer of nuts and drizzle them with the sriracha and honey. Use a silicone spatula to stir them well and fully distribute the flavourings. Cook for 3 more minutes, stirring the nuts halfway through.

3   You can serve these hot or cold. If I'm leaving them to cool down, I just leave them in the air fryer drawer on a heatproof surface, which allows them to crisp up. Once cooled, they may have clumped together, but you can easily break them apart before serving.

PER SERVING

CALORIES	FAT	SAT FAT	CARBS	SUGARS	FIBRE	PROTEIN	SALT
216	18G	3.2G	3.4G	2.3G	2.7G	9.5G	0.35G

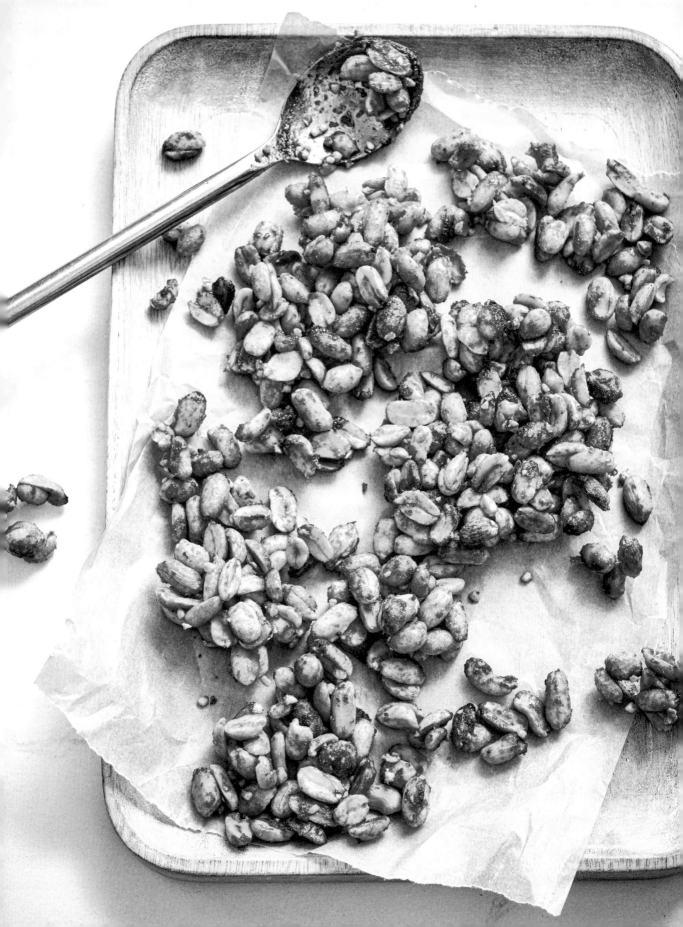

OXO ROAST POTATOES

SERVES 4
PREP TIME 15 minutes
COOK TIME 40 minutes

1kg (2lb 4oz) Maris Piper or other white floury potatoes, peeled and quartered (make sure the pieces are roughly equal-sized)

2 beef Oxo cubes, or equivalent (you need a stock cube you can finely crumble)

spray oil

These tasty roast potatoes come out of the air fryer crisp and delicious.

1 As you prepare the potatoes, drop them into a large saucepan of cold water. Once all the potatoes are prepared and in the pan, crumble in 1 Oxo cube.

2 Bring to the boil on the hob, then simmer for 5 minutes.

3 Preheat both air fryer drawers to 160°C (325°F).

4 After the potatoes have simmered for 5 minutes, drain them and leave to steam dry in a colander for a couple of minutes, shaking a couple of times.

5 Crumble up the remaining Oxo cube as finely as possible and sprinkle it over the potatoes, spray with oil and toss the potatoes a few times: you want to roughen up the outsides a little bit and also distribute the crumbled stock cube (make sure there aren't any big clumps).

6 Divide the potatoes between the drawers and cook for 30 minutes, shaking a couple of times during cooking to make sure they cook evenly.

7 After 30 minutes, increase the temperature to 200°C (400°F) and give them 5 minutes at the higher temperature. They should now be crisp on the outside and soft in the middle.

PER SERVING

CALORIES	FAT	SAT FAT	CARBS	SUGARS	FIBRE	PROTEIN	SALT
210	1.2G	0.1G	43G	1.8G	3.1G	5.3G	0.9G

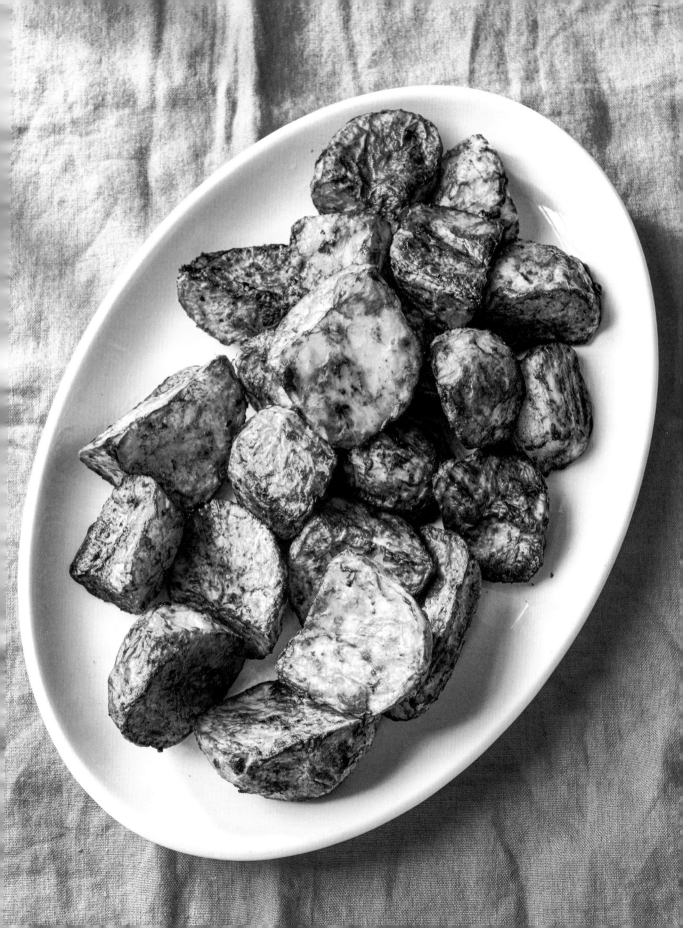

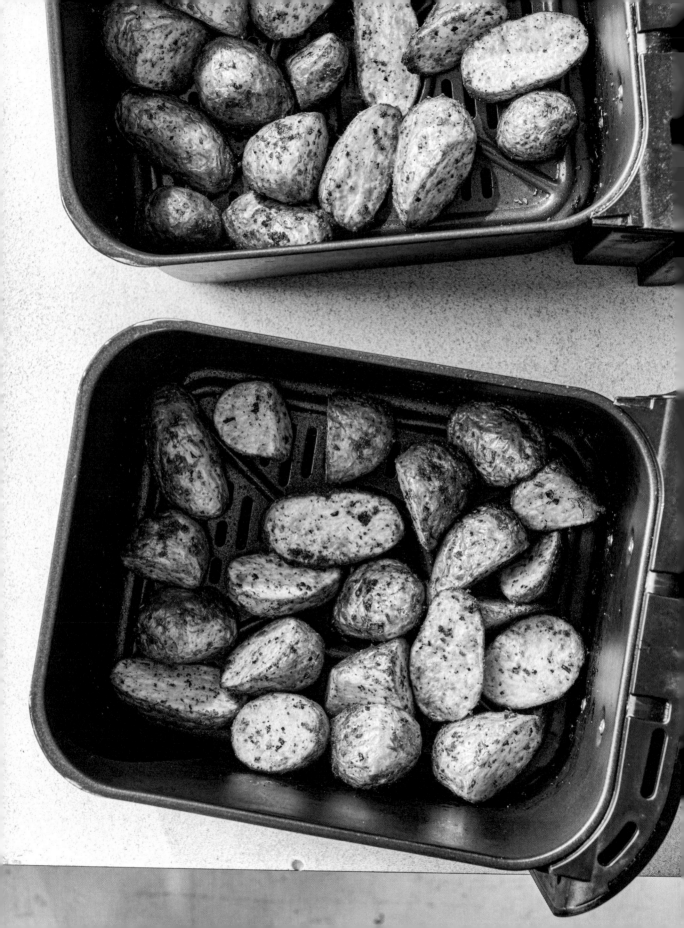

MINI ROSEMARY ROAST POTATOES

SERVES 4
PREP TIME 5 minutes
COOK TIME 20 minutes

900g (2lb) baby potatoes, halved if they are on the larger side

1 tablespoon olive oil

2 tablespoons finely chopped rosemary leaves (or the same amount of dried rosemary)

1 tablespoon garlic granules

1 teaspoon coarsely ground salt

½ teaspoon paprika

It's great to have an easy potato recipe which goes with most things, and these baby roasted potatoes are deliciously flavoured with a simple rosemary seasoning. They are perfect with Worcestershire Roast Beef (see page 104).

1   Preheat both air fryer drawers to 200°C (400°F).

2   Put the potatoes in a mixing bowl with the olive oil and mix until well coated. Add the rosemary, garlic granules, salt and paprika and stir again to coat the potatoes evenly.

3   Divide the potatoes between the 2 drawers and cook for 20 minutes, giving them a shake every 5 minutes to ensure even cooking. Check them at 15 minutes as you may not need the full 20 minutes (it depends on the size of the potatoes). They should be lovely and crisp on the outside and fork-tender in the middle: make sure you check the biggest one!

PER SERVING

CALORIES	FAT	SAT FAT	CARBS	SUGARS	FIBRE	PROTEIN	SALT
192	3.5G	0.6G	34G	3.2G	4.4G	4.2G	1.3G

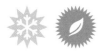

EASY ROASTED RATATOUILLE

SERVES 4
PREP TIME 15 minutes
COOK TIME 20–25 minutes

2 red onions, each cut into
   8 wedges

1 aubergine, chopped into 1cm
   (½ inch) pieces

2 courgettes, chopped into 2cm
   (¾ inch) pieces

2 red, orange or yellow peppers,
   deseeded and finely chopped

1 tablespoon olive oil

2 tablespoons balsamic vinegar

6 garlic cloves, thinly sliced

500g (1lb 2oz) tomato passata

1 tablespoon dried thyme

1 tablespoon dried rosemary

salt and pepper

I often make up a batch of this at the weekend to see me through some easy meals during the week. I serve it as a side to meat, fish or sausages, sometimes as a pasta sauce, as an extra portion of veg with whatever I'm eating for lunch, or sometimes blend the leftovers into a soup by adding some stock and extra canned tomatoes and herbs.

1   Remove the crisper plates and preheat both air fryer drawers to 200°C (400°F).

2   Put the red onion wedges in a mixing bowl and add the aubergine, courgettes and peppers, then the olive oil and balsamic vinegar and mix well. Divide the vegetable mixture between the 2 air fryer drawers and cook for 15 minutes, stirring every 5 minutes. After 10 minutes, stir in the garlic slices.

3   After 15 minutes, divide the passata and the dried herbs between the 2 drawers, season with salt and pepper, stir and cook for another 5 minutes.

4   Try a piece of the aubergine to check that the consistency is to your liking. If you'd like it a little softer, cook it for another 5 minutes and try it again. The ratatouille is now ready to serve, or store in an airtight container for when you need it. Once fully cooled, it will keep in the refrigerator for up to 5 days.

PER SERVING

CALORIES	FAT	SAT FAT	CARBS	SUGARS	FIBRE	PROTEIN	SALT
172	4.2G	0.6G	22G	19G	6.4G	5/9G	0.2G

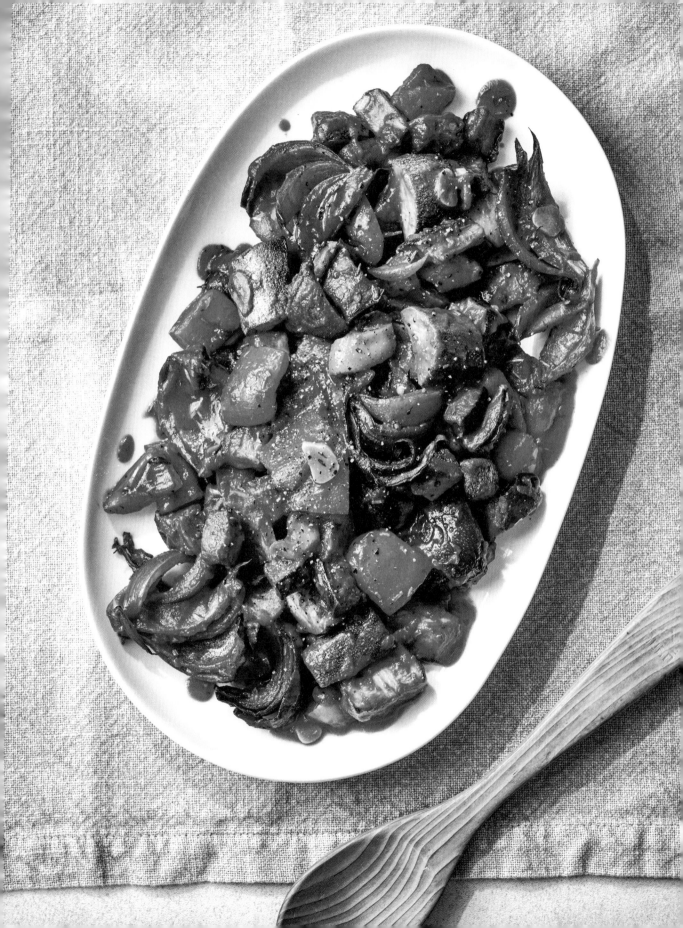

GOLDEN CHIPPIES

SERVES 4
PREP TIME 15 minutes
COOK TIME 20–25 minutes

900g (2lb) potatoes, peeled and
cut into 1cm (½ inch) cubes
1 teaspoon onion granules
1 teaspoon garlic granules
1 teaspoon ground turmeric
½ teaspoon salt
1 tablespoon olive oil

Crisp on the outside and tender in the middle, these seasoned potato cubes, infused with garlic, onion and turmeric, make for a deliciously satisfying side dish.

1 Preheat both air fryer drawers to 195°C (385°F).

2 In a large bowl, mix the potato cubes, onion and garlic granules, turmeric and salt, then stir in the oil thoroughly.

3 Divide the potatoes equally between the 2 drawers, then cook for 20–25 minutes, until the potatoes are crisp and golden on the outside and soft in the middle.

PER SERVING

CALORIES	FAT	SAT FAT	CARBS	SUGARS	FIBRE	PROTEIN	SALT
214	3.4G	0.5G	39G	1.9G	3G	4.8G	0.62G

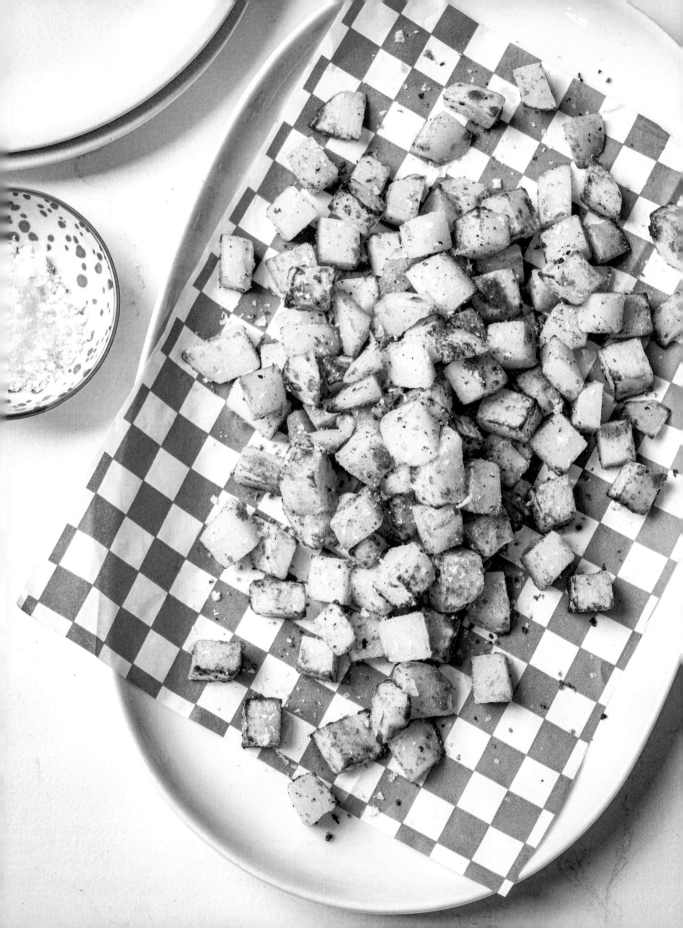

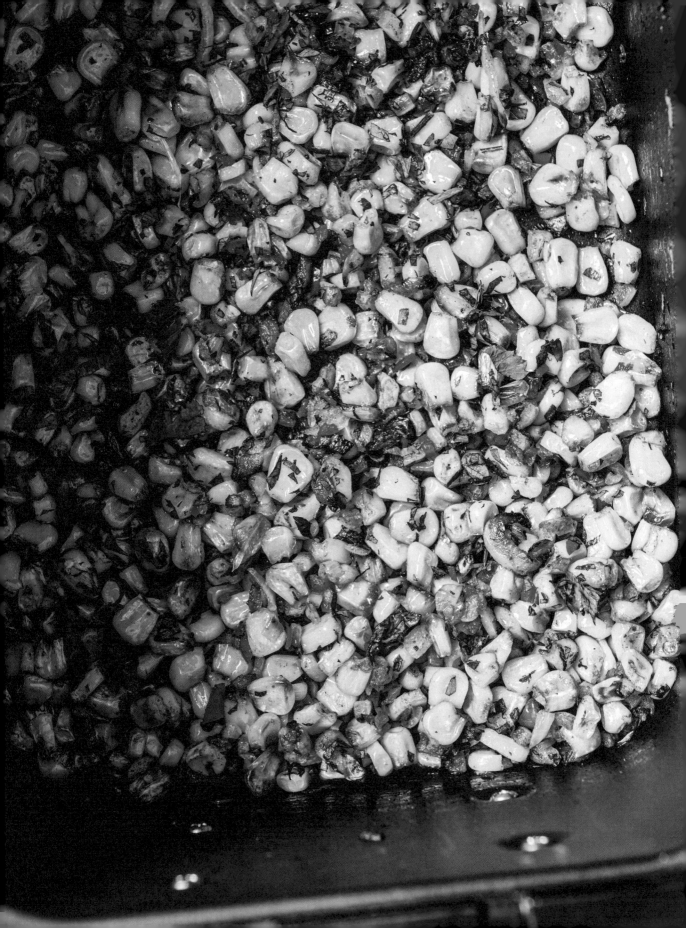

SOUTHWESTERN CORN SALAD

SERVES 4
PREP TIME 10 minutes
COOK TIME 15 minutes

300g (10½oz) frozen sweetcorn

1 onion, finely chopped

1 tablespoon pickled jalapeños, chopped

1 red pepper, deseeded and finely chopped

1 teaspoon olive oil

1 teaspoon ground cumin

juice of 1 lemon

handful of parsley leaves, finely chopped

½ teaspoon salt

I find a corn salad makes such a colourful and tasty side to all sorts of dishes, and this one will go with many of the recipes in this book. Try it with Hunter's Chicken, Chipotle Chicken Burgers with Garlic-lime Sauce or Worcestershire Roast Beef (see pages 96, 116 and 151).

1 Remove the crisper plates and preheat both air fryer drawers to 200°C (400°F).

2 In a mixing bowl, combine the sweetcorn, onion, jalapeños, red pepper, olive oil, cumin and 1 tablespoon of the lemon juice. Divide the mixture equally between the 2 drawers, spreading it into an even layer, and cook for 15 minutes, stirring every 5 minutes.

3 Return the mixture to the bowl, stir in the remaining lemon juice, the chopped parsley and salt, and serve, hot or cold.

PER SERVING

CALORIES	FAT	SAT FAT	CARBS	SUGARS	FIBRE	PROTEIN	SALT
131	2.4G	0.4G	22G	8.2G	3.2G	3.4G	0.82G

FRIED EDAMAME

SERVES 4
PREP TIME 2 minutes
COOK TIME 12 minutes

200g (7oz) frozen edamame (no need to defrost)
1 teaspoon sesame oil
½ teaspoon coarsely ground salt
1 teaspoon garlic granules

These beans are great as a side, snack or scattered over stir-fries or salads.

1 Remove the crisper plate from 1 drawer of the air fryer and preheat that drawer to 200°C (400°F).

2 In a bowl, mix the edamame, oil, salt and garlic granules and transfer to the preheated air fryer drawer. Cook for 12 minutes, giving the drawer a shake a couple of times during cooking.

PER SERVING

CALORIES	FAT	SAT FAT	CARBS	SUGARS	FIBRE	PROTEIN	SALT
66	3.4G	0.2G	2.2G	1.4G	2.5G	5.2G	0.62G

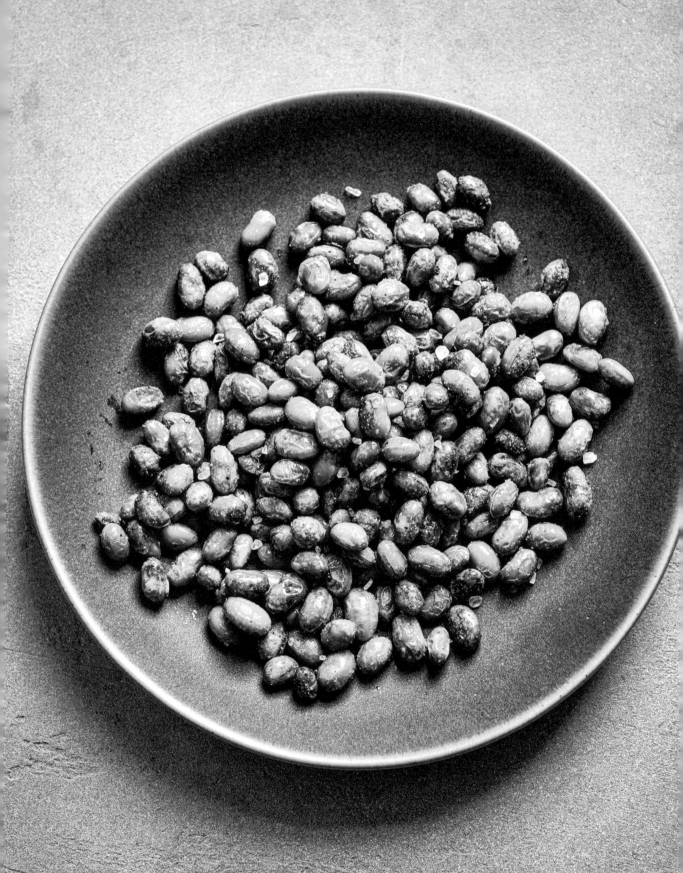

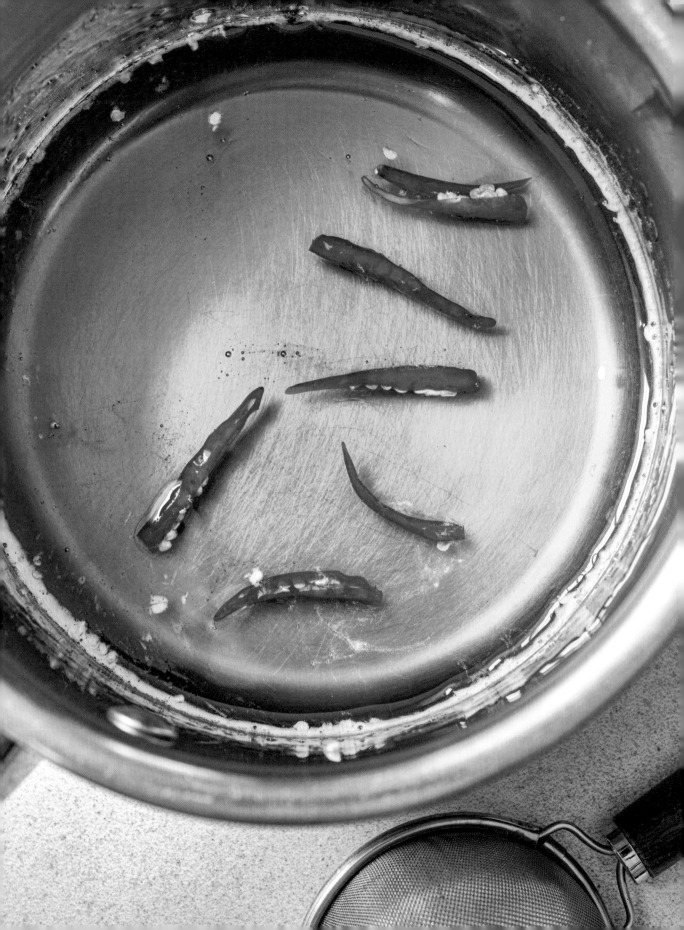

HOT HONEY

MAKES 1 small jar / **SERVES** 12
PREP TIME 5 minutes, plus steeping time
COOK TIME 2 minutes

250ml (9fl oz) honey
4 birds eye chillies, stalks removed and halved
1 tablespoon apple cider vinegar

Okay, so this one isn't made in an air fryer, but it does go perfectly with many of the meals that come out of the air fryer (just try it with Chipotle Chicken Burgers with Garlic-lime Sauce, see page 116), as well as making a tasty drizzle or dip for just about anything (salads, rice, meat, pizza, chips), so I thoroughly recommend giving it a go!

1   Put the honey in a small pan with the chillies and bring up to a gentle simmer. Simmer for 2 minutes, then remove from the heat and leave to steep for 15 minutes.

2   Stir through the vinegar, then remove the chillies and transfer the honey to a clean jar.

3   This should keep for 3–6 months in the refrigerator, but watch out for signs of spoilage, such as visible mould, or an unpleasant smell or colour, and discard it.

PER SERVING

CALORIES	FAT	SAT FAT	CARBS	SUGARS	FIBRE	PROTEIN	SALT
91	0	0	23	23	0	0	0

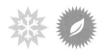

REFRIED BEANS

SERVES 6
PREP TIME 5 minutes
COOK TIME 15 minutes

1 tablespoon olive oil
1 small onion, finely chopped
1 teaspoon coarsely ground salt
2 garlic cloves, crushed
½ teaspoon chilli powder
¼ teaspoon ground cumin
2 x 400g (14oz) cans of pinto
  beans, drained and rinsed
150ml (¼ pint) boiling water
juice of 1 lime

I love refried beans, and this air fryer version is perfect in fajitas, burritos or with Mexican-inspired rice bowls or chilli con carne.

1   Remove the crisper plate from 1 air fryer drawer, add the oil and preheat the drawer to 200°C (400°F).

2   Add the onion and salt, give it a stir, then cook for 5 minutes, stirring halfway through.

3   Stir through the garlic, chilli and cumin, then add the pinto beans and stir again. Cook for 5 minutes, stirring halfway through.

4   Pour in the boiling water, stir well and cook for another 5 minutes.

5   Use a silicone potato masher to mash the beans, then stir well. They should have a creamy, thick consistency. If you do not have a silicone masher, transfer the beans to a bowl before mashing so that you don't scratch the nonstick surface of the drawer. Stir in the lime juice before serving.

PER SERVING

CALORIES	FAT	SAT FAT	CARBS	SUGARS	FIBRE	PROTEIN	SALT
109	2.8G	0.4G	11G	1.8G	6G	6.3G	0.87G

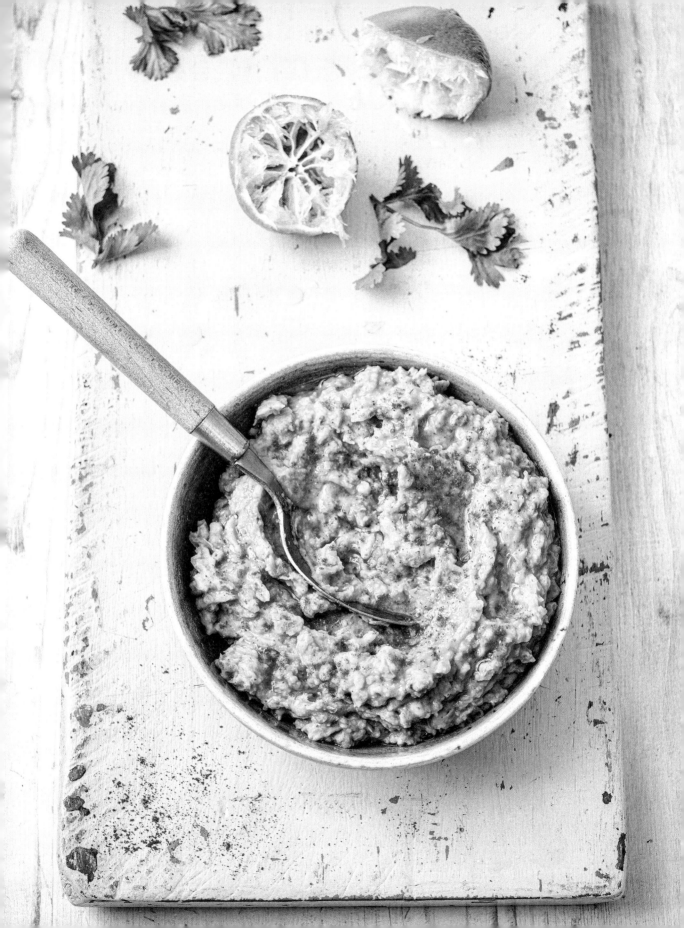

PERFECT CHIPS

SERVES 4
PREP TIME 25 minutes
COOK TIME 24 minutes

900g (2lb) white floury potatoes
  (I usually use Maris Piper)
spray oil
coarsely ground salt

If you haven't already cracked how to make great air fryer chips, here's how I do it. It might not be rocket science, but it's imperative to be able to make lovely crispy chips in an air fryer!

1   Peel the potatoes and cut them into evenly sized chips. Place in a large bowl of cold water and leave to soak for 20 minutes.

2   Drain them, shaking as you go to remove as much water as possible, spread them out over a chopping board or similar and pat them dry with kitchen paper or a clean tea towel. Now place them in a large bowl and spray with oil; toss and spray again, repeating this until all the chips have been lightly coated with oil.

3   Preheat both air fryer drawers to 160°C (325°F) and divide the chips equally between them, shaking so that they lie in a single layer. Cook for 12 minutes, shaking halfway through.

4   Now increase the temperature of the air fryer to 200°C (400°F) and cook the chips for a further 12–15 minutes, again shaking halfway through, but keep an eye on them towards the end of the cooking time. They should be cooked through by now, so you are just trying to achieve your preferred level of crispness and colour. If you aren't quite happy with how browned they are, cook a little more and check on them at 2-minute intervals.

5   Once they are cooked to perfection, place them in a bowl, season with salt and toss to coat.

PER SERVING

CALORIES	FAT	SAT FAT	CARBS	SUGARS	FIBRE	PROTEIN	SALT
183	0.7G	TRACE	38G	1.6G	2.7G	4.5G	0.25G

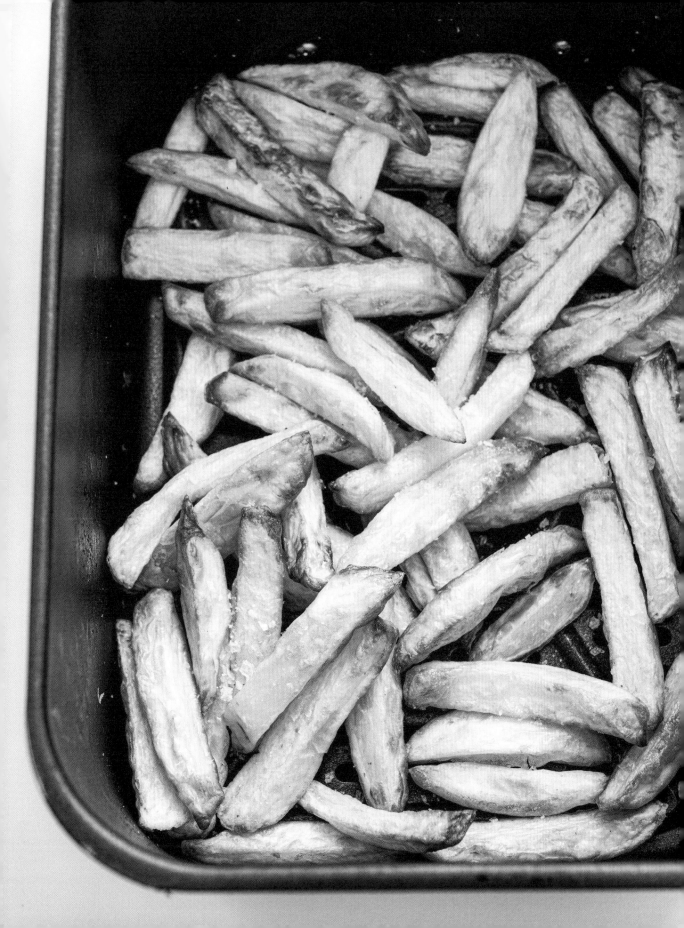

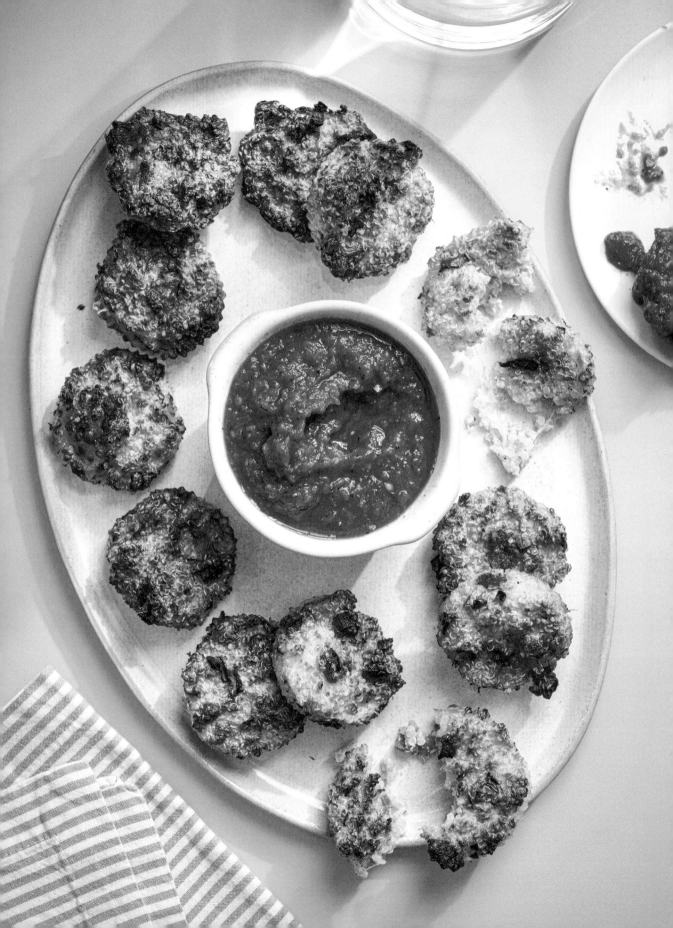

SPICY PIZZA POPS

MAKES 18
PREP TIME 10 minutes
COOK TIME 45 minutes

100g (3½oz) quinoa (uncooked weight)

140g (5oz) mozzarella cheese, finely chopped

30g (1oz) chorizo, finely chopped

30g (1oz) pickled jalapeños, finely chopped

1 egg, lightly beaten

spray oil

salt and pepper

FOR THE DIPPING SAUCE

400g (14oz) can of good-quality chopped tomatoes (my favourite brand is Mutti)

1 tablespoon tomato purée

1 garlic clove

1 teaspoon dried oregano

1 teaspoon dried basil

½ teaspoon onion granules

½ teaspoon coarsely ground salt

Golden baked pizza-style bites are crispy on the outside and filled with chorizo, mozzarella and jalapeño. These make a satisfying snack dipped into a simple tomato sauce.

1 Cook the quinoa according to the packet instructions then leave to cool slightly while you prepare the rest of the ingredients.

2 In a mixing bowl, combine the quinoa (make sure it's fully drained and not piping hot), mozzarella, chorizo, jalapeños, salt and pepper and stir well to combine. Add the beaten egg and mix this through.

3 Lay out 18 silicone cupcake cases and add about 1 tablespoon of mixture to each case. Spray the tops with oil.

4 Preheat both air fryer drawers to 200°C (400°F).

5 Place the cupcake cases in the drawers (you will be able to fit about 8 in each one, so will need to cook these pops in 2 batches), then cook for 15 minutes, until fully cooked through, golden brown, and crisp on top and around the edges – you might need to give them a few more minutes if necessary.

6 Meanwhile, make the sauce. Put all the ingredients into a food processor or blender (or use a stick blender) and blend into a smooth sauce.

7 Serve the pizza pops alongside the sauce in a dipping bowl.

PER SERVING

CALORIES	FAT	SAT FAT	CARBS	SUGARS	FIBRE	PROTEIN	SALT
58	2.9G	1.4G	4.1G	1.4G	0.8G	3.4G	0.41G

BISCOFF FLAPJACKS

LITTLE OATY APPLE CRUMBLES

BUTTERY CINNAMON-VANILLA
APPLES

5-MINUTE CHOCOLATE BROWNIES

ROAST GRAPE CLAFOUTIS

MERINGUE NEST S'MORES

STICKY STUFFED STONE FRUIT

MARS BABY BAKES

STRAWBERRY AND PISTACHIO
SCONES

SMALL BATCH CHOCOLATE CHIP
COOKIES

WELSH CAKES

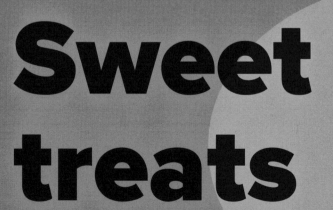

Sweet treats

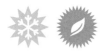

BISCOFF FLAPJACKS

MAKES 16
PREP TIME 20 minutes
COOK TIME 35 minutes

100g (3½oz) caramelized biscuit spread, such as Biscoff, plus 1 tablespoon for drizzling

80g (2¾oz) honey

50g (1¾oz) butter

350g (12oz) porridge oats (not jumbo oats)

2 eggs

These flapjacks are soft-baked with a crunchy top and a delicious Biscoff twist. They have a much lower sugar content than you'll find in most flapjack recipes, but they are still totally delicious and are super-easy to make when you need a freshly baked treat.

1   In a saucepan, melt together the Biscoff spread, honey and butter until liquid and fully combined.

2   Measure the oats into a mixing bowl and pour over the Biscoff mixture, using a spatula to get it all out of the pan. Mix thoroughly, then leave to cool for 5 minutes.

3   Remove the crisper plate from 1 air fryer drawer and preheat that drawer to 160°C (325°F).

4   Beat the eggs, then mix them into the slightly cooled flapjack mixture until thoroughly combined.

5   Carefully line the hot drawer with nonstick baking paper, tip in the flapjack mixture and use a spatula to press it down in an even layer in the drawer. Cook for 25 minutes.

6   Carefully lift the flapjack out of the drawer and leave to cool for at least 15 minutes.

7   In a small bowl, melt the 1 tablespoon of Biscoff spread in the microwave (this should take 45–60 seconds). Drizzle it over the top of the flapjack, spread evenly using the back of a teaspoon, then leave to fully cool and set. Once cold, cut into 16 equal pieces.

PER SERVING

CALORIES	FAT	SAT FAT	CARBS	SUGARS	FIBRE	PROTEIN	SALT
182	7.9G	2.7G	23G	6.6G	1.9G	3.9G	0.13G

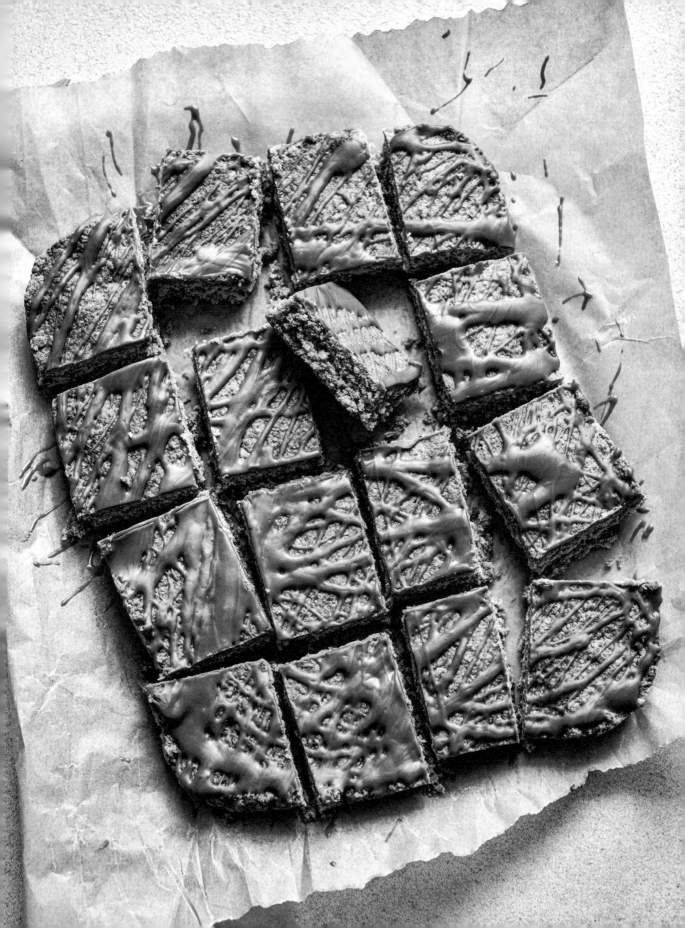

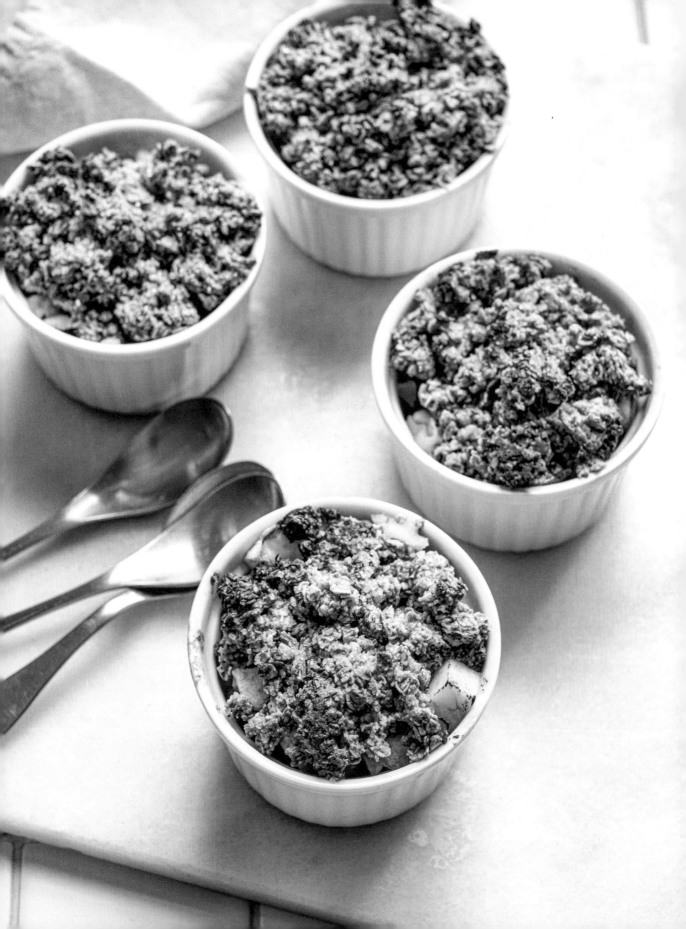

LITTLE OATY APPLE CRUMBLES

MAKES 4
PREP TIME 10 minutes
COOK TIME 21 minutes

2 cooking apples (total weight about 450g / 1lb), peeled, cored and chopped
1 teaspoon vanilla extract
100ml (3½fl oz) water

FOR THE CRUMBLE
80g (2¾oz) oats
1 tablespoon plain flour
1 tablespoon honey
½ teaspoon ground cinnamon
1 egg, lightly beaten
2 teaspoons demerara sugar

Perfectly tender apples topped with a crunchy oat crumble, this is a quick and easy dessert to cook in the air fryer.

1 Preheat both air fryer drawers to 175°C (347°F).

2 In a bowl, mix together the apples, vanilla extract and measured water. Divide the mixture between 4 ramekins.

3 In another bowl, mix the oats and flour with the honey, cinnamon and egg. Divide this crumble mixture between the 4 ramekins to top the apple, then sprinkle ½ teaspoon demerara sugar over the top of each.

4 Cover each ramekin with foil, tucking it under so it doesn't fly off in the air fryer. Place in the drawers and air fry for 18 minutes, until the apples are tender.

5 Carefully remove the foil, then return the crumbles to air fry for another 3 minutes to brown the topping.

PER SERVING

CALORIES	FAT	SAT FAT	CARBS	SUGARS	FIBRE	PROTEIN	SALT
194	3.3G	0.7G	34G	16G	3.8G	5G	TRACE

BUTTERY CINNAMON-VANILLA APPLES

SERVES 4
PREP TIME 10 minutes
COOK TIME 10 minutes

Sweet, buttery, tender apples combined with sugar cinnamon and vanilla are a little taste of autumn, but can be enjoyed all year round! Serve these with hot custard, a scoop of vanilla ice cream or simply some Greek yogurt.

2 tablespoons (30g / 1oz) unsalted butter, melted

1½ tablespoons demerara sugar

1 teaspoon ground cinnamon

½ teaspoon vanilla extract

pinch of salt

4 tart apples, such as Granny Smiths, cored and cut into thin wedges

spray oil

1 Remove the crisper plates and preheat both air fryer drawers to 190°C (375°F).

2 In a small bowl, combine the melted butter, sugar, cinnamon, vanilla extract and salt.

3 Place the apple wedges in a large bowl and pour over the butter mixture. Stir well to ensure that all the apple is coated.

4 Spray a little oil into the preheated air fryer drawers and tip in the apple slices, spreading them into single layers. Cook for 10 minutes, shaking the drawers halfway through the cooking time. After 10 minutes, the apples should be tender and caramelized.

5 Serve however you fancy!

PER SERVING

CALORIES	FAT	SAT FAT	CARBS	SUGARS	FIBRE	PROTEIN	SALT
168	7.3G	3.9G	23G	23G	3.9G	0.8G	0.62G

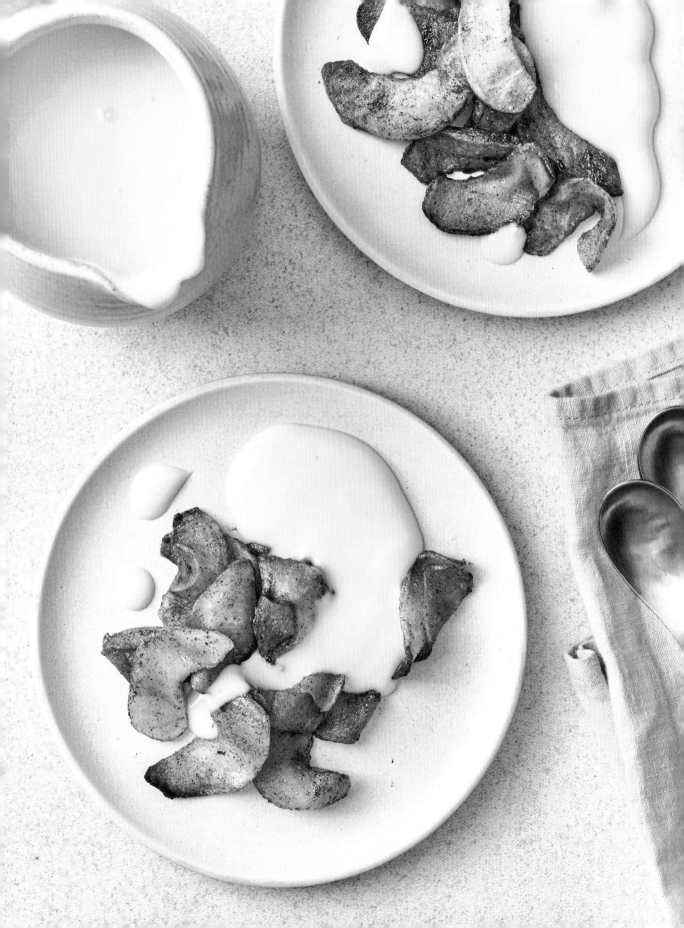

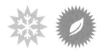

5-MINUTE CHOCOLATE BROWNIES

MAKES 8
PREP TIME 5 minutes
COOK TIME 15 minutes

150g (5½oz) chocolate hazelnut spread, such as Nutella

2 eggs, lightly beaten

1 teaspoon vanilla extract

1 tablespoon dark brown sugar

75g (2¾oz) plain flour

15g (½oz) cocoa powder

¼ teaspoon table salt

100g (3½oz) mixed chocolate chips (milk and white)

spray oil

Brownies are my girls' favourite treat, and this is a very popular recipe, partly because they are so quick to make! My kids can easily bake them without help. You will need a baking dish or tin that fits into your air fryer drawers. I have found that medium (215 x 158mm / 8 x 6 inch) foil takeaway containers are great for this (and can be reused). You may need to lengthen the timings here if you are using a ceramic or silicone dish.

1   Preheat 1 air fryer drawer to 180°C (350°F).

2   In a mixing bowl, beat together the chocolate spread and eggs with the vanilla extract and sugar until well combined. Add the flour, cocoa powder and salt and fold in to form a batter. Stir through the chocolate chips.

3   Choose a medium foil container or baking dish / tin that fits snugly in the air fryer drawer (see recipe introduction) and spray it with cooking oil. Scrape the batter into the container and make sure it's evenly distributed.

4   Place in the air fryer drawer and cook for 15 minutes. The top should be glossy with a slight crispness and the brownie should be cooked through. If you give it a little wobble and it still seems too wet, give it a few more minutes.

5   Allow to cool for at least 10 minutes before cutting into 8 pieces.

PER BROWNIE

CALORIES	FAT	SAT FAT	CARBS	SUGARS	FIBRE	PROTEIN	SALT
234	12G	4.9G	26G	19G	1G	5.2G	0.23G

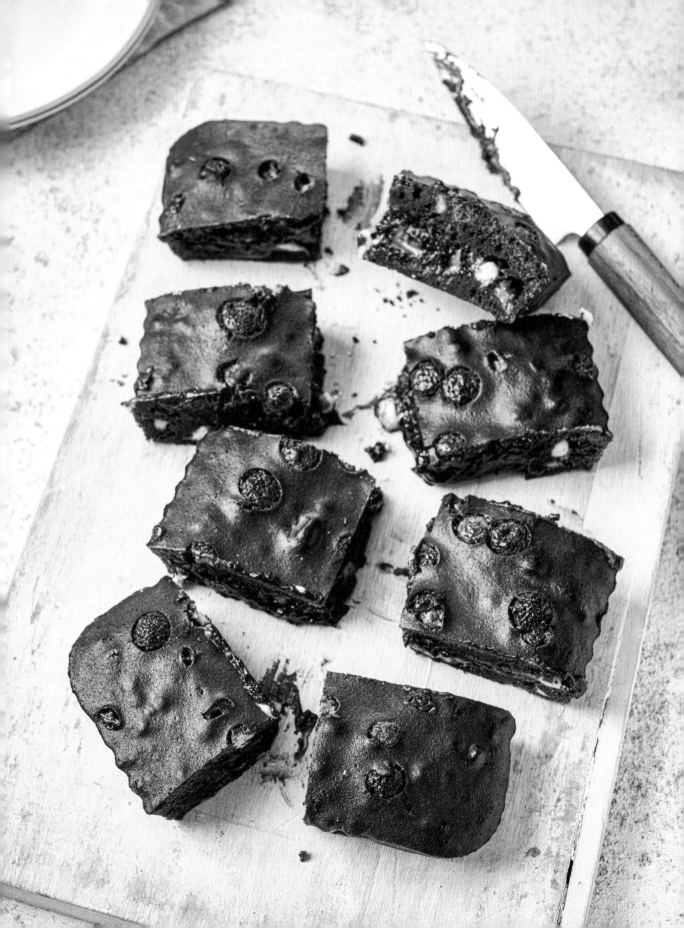

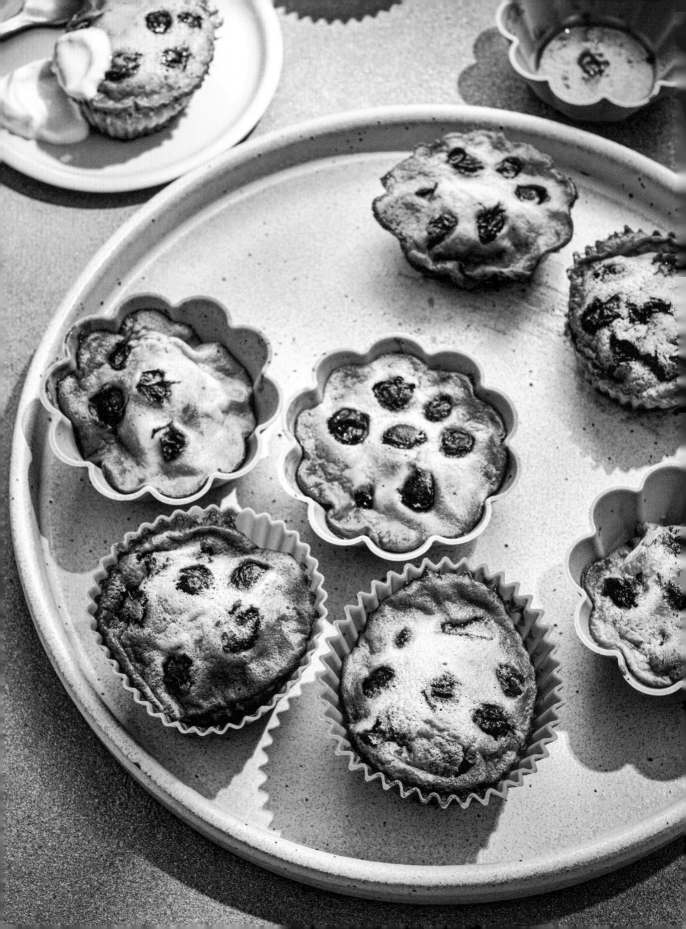

ROAST GRAPE CLAFOUTIS

MAKES 8
PREP TIME 5 minutes
COOK TIME 12 minutes

spray oil

150g (5½oz) small purple grapes, ideally Sable

1 tablespoon honey

¼ teaspoon balsamic vinegar

2 eggs

120ml (4fl oz) milk

60g (2¼oz) caster sugar

½ teaspoon vanilla extract

60g (2¼oz) plain flour

Essentially little baked custards, these puddings work really well with small and intensely flavoured grapes, such as Sable.

1   Lightly spray 8 silicone cupcake cases with oil. Preheat both air fryer drawers to 200°C (400°F).

2   Place the grapes in a bowl and mix them with the honey and vinegar so they are well covered. Divide the grapes between the cupcake cases, place in the air fryer and cook for 5 minutes, until their skins have started to split and they've released a little juice.

3   Meanwhile, whisk the eggs, milk, sugar and vanilla in a bowl until well combined. Add the flour, a little at a time, and fold in until you have a smooth batter.

4   When the grapes are done, reduce the temperature of both air fryer drawers to 160°C (325°F). Divide the batter between the cupcake cases in the drawers, spooning or pouring it directly on to the grapes. Cook for 12 minutes, until puffed up. Allow to cool for a couple of minutes before serving as they are, or with a blob of yogurt.

PER SERVING

CALORIES	FAT	SAT FAT	CARBS	SUGARS	FIBRE	PROTEIN	SALT
105	1.8G	0.6G	19G	13G	0.5G	3.1G	TRACE

MERINGUE NEST S'MORES

SERVES 4
PREP TIME 2 minutes
COOK TIME 4 minutes

40g (1½oz) milk chocolate chips
4 meringue nests
8 marshmallows, cut in half

These are a life-saver when you want a quick, simple and fun pudding. We make them when my girls have friends over, or sometimes just on those 'Is there anything for pudding?' days.

1 Preheat both air fryer drawers to 180°C (350°F).

2 Place 10g (½oz) chocolate chips in each meringue nest, then lay 4 halves of marshmallow in a circle over the top. They should be sticky enough to lightly adhere to the meringue.

3 Place 2 nests in each air fryer drawer and cook for 4 minutes. By this time the marshmallows should have puffed up, be melted on the inside and slightly browned on top. The chocolate chips should also have melted.

4 Use a spatula to lift out each meringue nest. Be careful here as the meringue is fragile, but if you scoop it up gently with a spatula, it should hold together.

PER SERVING

CALORIES	FAT	SAT FAT	CARBS	SUGARS	FIBRE	PROTEIN	SALT
156	3.2G	1.9G	30G	27G	0G	2G	TRACE

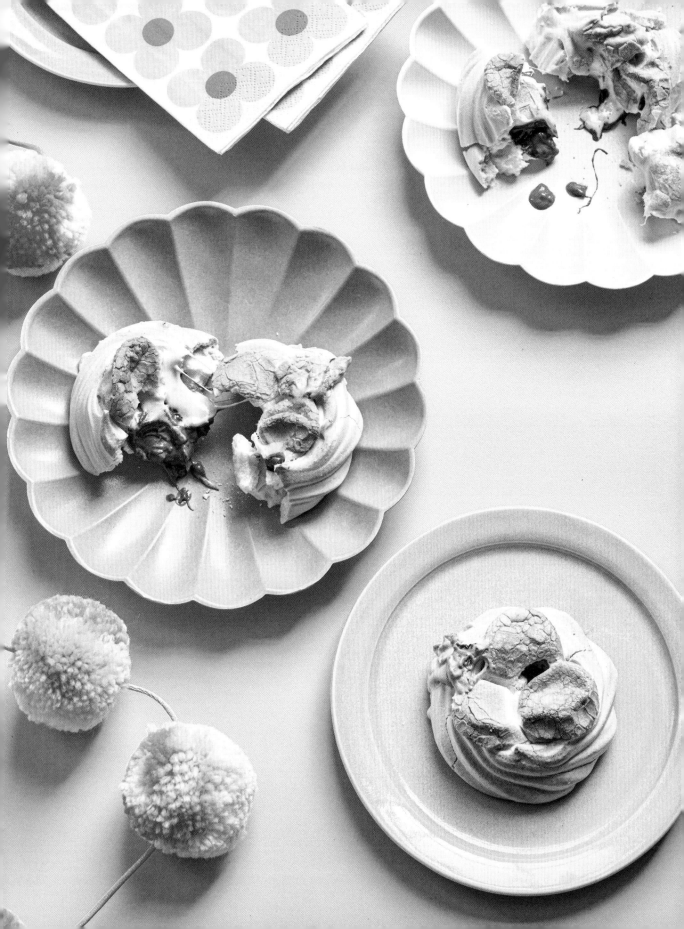

STICKY STUFFED STONE FRUIT

SERVES 6 generously (2 halves per person), or 12 more lightly
PREP TIME 15 minutes
COOK TIME 12 minutes

6 peaches or nectarines
2 tablespoons maple syrup
100g (3½oz) ground almonds
1 egg, lightly beaten
½ teaspoon almond extract
2 teaspoons caster sugar
pinch of salt
1 tablespoon lemon juice

These are lovely served hot from the air fryer with a scoop of frozen yogurt. These would make a super-easy dessert if you were hosting a dinner party.

1   Slice the fruits in half and remove the stones. Place in a bowl and toss with 1 tablespoon of the maple syrup.

2   In a bowl, combine the ground almonds with the egg, almond extract, remaining 1 tablespoon maple syrup, the sugar, pinch of salt and the lemon juice, and mix well. Spoon a generous amount of mixture into the fruit cavities.

3   Preheat both air fryer drawers to 160°C (325°F). Carefully line the hot drawers with nonstick baking paper and place the fruit halves inside, stuffed side up, then cook for 12 minutes.

PER SERVING

CALORIES	FAT	SAT FAT	CARBS	SUGARS	FIBRE	PROTEIN	SALT
178	10G	1G	14G	12G	3.6G	5.7G	1.3G

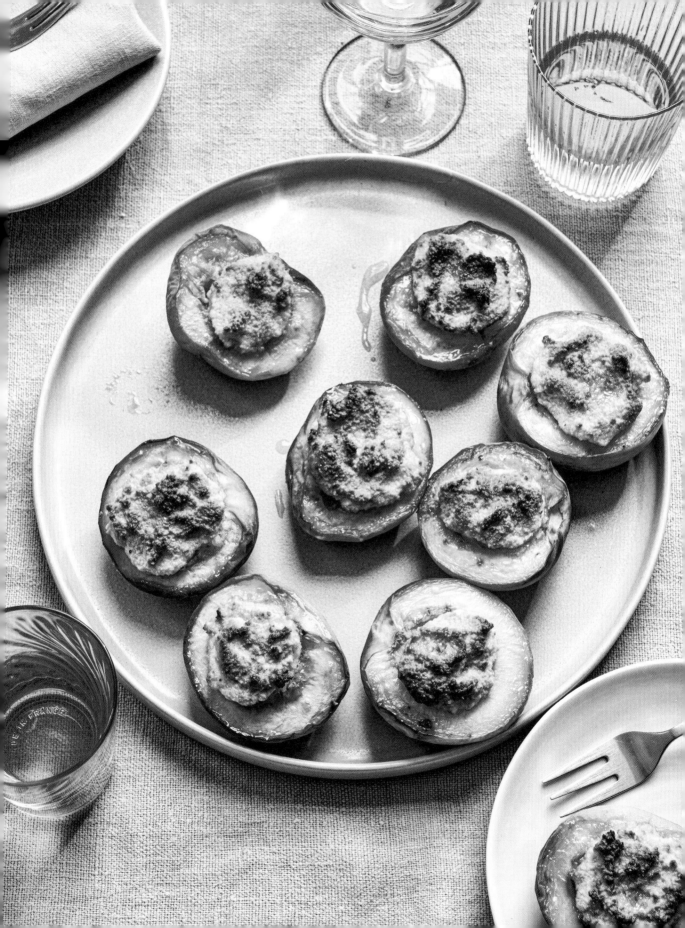

MARS BABY BAKES

MAKES 6
PREP TIME 10 minutes
COOK TIME 10 minutes

---

1 puff pastry sheet, 24cm
(9½ inches) long
1 Mars bar (51g / 1¾oz), cut into
6 equal pieces

Channelling a deep-fried Mars bar, these are little bites of puff pastry filled with melty Mars. I don't think anyone could call them healthy, but they are a fun, small treat that the kids can help with.

1 Unroll the pastry sheet. Cut a 10cm (4 inch) strip off the pastry length to leave you with a 24 x 10cm (9½ x 4 inch) long piece (save the rest of the pastry for another recipe). Cut the pastry strip into 6 pieces, each 4cm (1½ inches) wide. Now cut each piece in half lengthways – you should end up with 12 small rectangles measuring 5 x 4cm (2 x 1½ inches).

2 Sandwich each slice of Mars bar between 2 pieces of pastry and use a fork to indent and seal all around the edges to form neat little parcels.

3 Preheat both air fryer drawers to 170°C (340°F).

4 Lay a piece of baking paper in the bottom of each drawer and place 3 baby bakes in each, with a little space between them. Cook for 10 minutes, by which time the pastry should be puffed and golden brown and the Mars inside melted and gooey. Enjoy while warm.

PER BAKE

CALORIES	FAT	SAT FAT	CARBS	SUGARS	FIBRE	PROTEIN	SALT
129	17G	3.3G	12G	5.4G	0.6G	1.5G	0.21G

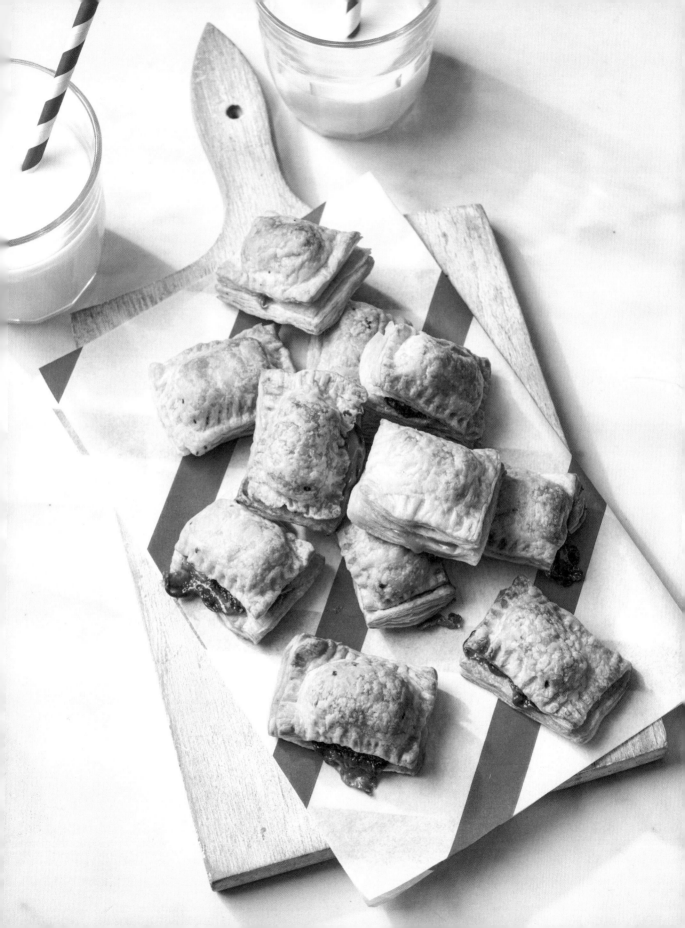

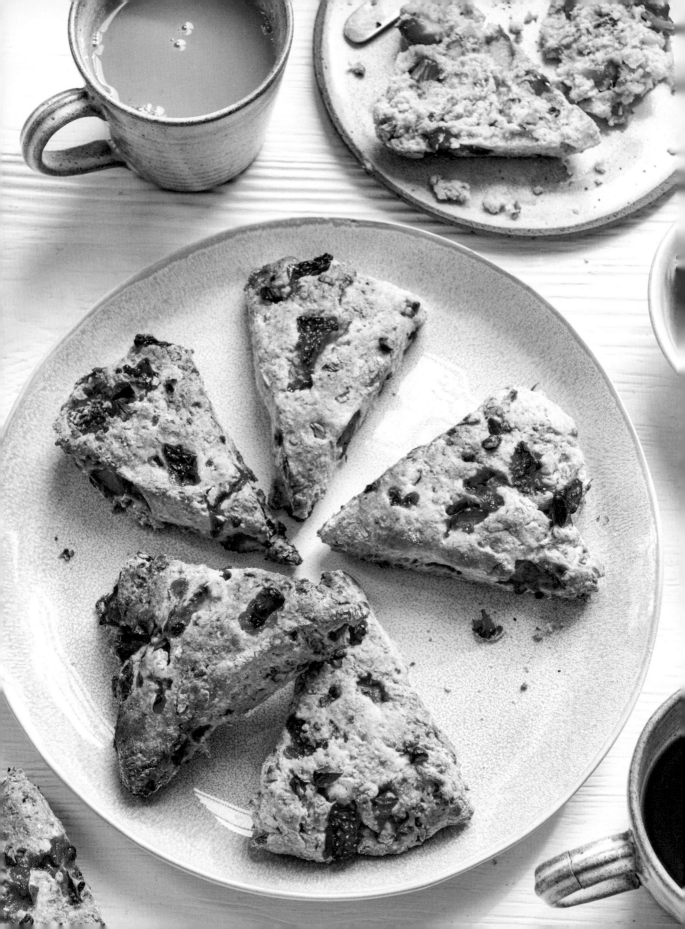

STRAWBERRY AND PISTACHIO SCONES

MAKES 8
PREP TIME 20 minutes
COOK TIME 12 minutes

250g (9oz) plain flour, plus more to dust

2 teaspoons baking powder

1 tablespoon caster sugar

pinch of salt

25g (1oz) butter, cut into small pieces

30g (1oz) fat-free Greek yogurt

1 egg

50ml (1¾fl oz) semi-skimmed milk, plus more if needed

1 teaspoon vanilla extract

150g (5½oz) strawberries, chopped

40g (1½oz) shelled unsalted pistachio nuts, crushed

Not much can beat a freshly baked scone, and these have the delicious flavour of strawberries with a satisfying pistachio crunch. You can spread them with jam, butter, cream, a combination of all three, or even pistachio spread if you're feeling fancy!

1 Put the flour in a mixing bowl with the baking powder, caster sugar and salt. Add the butter and yogurt. Use your fingers to rub the butter and yogurt into the flour, breaking down any lumps and bringing the flour to a crumb-like consistency.

2 Break the egg into a measuring jug and add the milk and vanilla extract. Beat together using a fork or small whisk.

3 Add the chopped strawberries and crushed pistachios to the dry flour mix and stir through. Pour in most of the egg mixture (reserve a small amount to brush over the scones later), then use a table knife to bring the wet and dry ingredients together to form a dough (you can use your hands for this once the wet ingredients have mostly combined with the dry). Form the dough into a ball (if it's too sticky just add a little more flour; if it's too dry, add a splash more milk).

4 On a lightly floured surface, lightly press down the dough into a flatter, round shape, about 3cm (1¼ inches) thick.

5 Preheat both air fryer drawers to 190°C (375°F).

6 Score the dough with a knife to mark out 8 equal pieces (like cutting a pizza), then use a sharp knife to cut out the 8 triangles. Transfer to the air fryer drawers (4 in each, spaced so they are not touching), brush with the remaining egg mix using a pastry brush, then cook for 12 minutes.

7 After this time, the scones should have risen, be a rich golden brown on top and cooked through. These are delicious warm or cold.

PER SCONE

CALORIES	FAT	SAT FAT	CARBS	SUGARS	FIBRE	PROTEIN	SALT
197	6.6G	2.4G	27G	3.6G	2.4G	5.7G	0.46G

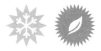

SMALL-BATCH CHOCOLATE CHIP COOKIES

MAKES 4
PREP TIME 10 minutes
COOK TIME 11 minutes

30g (1oz) butter, softened but not melted

30g (1oz) dark brown sugar

1 tablespoon caster sugar

1 egg yolk

½ teaspoon vanilla extract

50g (1¾oz) plain flour

pinch of bicarbonate of soda

50g (1¾oz) milk or dark chocolate chips, or cooking chocolate, cut into small chunks

The air fryer is perfect for making a small batch of delicious chocolate chip cookies with a beautiful crisp top and a chewy middle. My daughters and I have experimented with lots of recipes, and these were declared the best we had made. Just making four at a time works for me, as it means I'm not tempted to overindulge, but can still enjoy a freshly baked cookie.

1   Use a fork to cream together the butter, brown sugar and caster sugar. Add the egg yolk and vanilla extract and beat into the butter and sugar. Add the flour and bicarbonate of soda and mix through to form a dough. Add in most of the chocolate chips, reserving some to dot over the tops.

2   Preheat both air fryer drawers to 160°C (325°F).

3   Divide the mixture roughly into 4, then roll each piece into a ball. Slightly flatten each ball, then dot the top with the remaining chocolate chips.

4   Cut 2 pieces of nonstick baking paper and use to line the bottom of the hot air fryer drawers. Place the cookie balls inside, giving each as much space as you can, allowing them room to spread on all sides. Cook for 11 minutes, by which time the top of the cookies should be golden brown and slightly crisp. If you think they need a little longer, cook in further 1-minute increments until you are happy.

5   Remove the air fryer drawers and set them on a heatproof surface to allow the cookies to cool for 5 minutes. They will be very soft at first, so may fall apart if you try to remove them from the drawers straight away. Eat the cookies warm or cold.

PER COOKIE

CALORIES	FAT	SAT FAT	CARBS	SUGARS	FIBRE	PROTEIN	SALT
224	12G	6.6G	27G	18G	0.6G	2.9G	0.26G

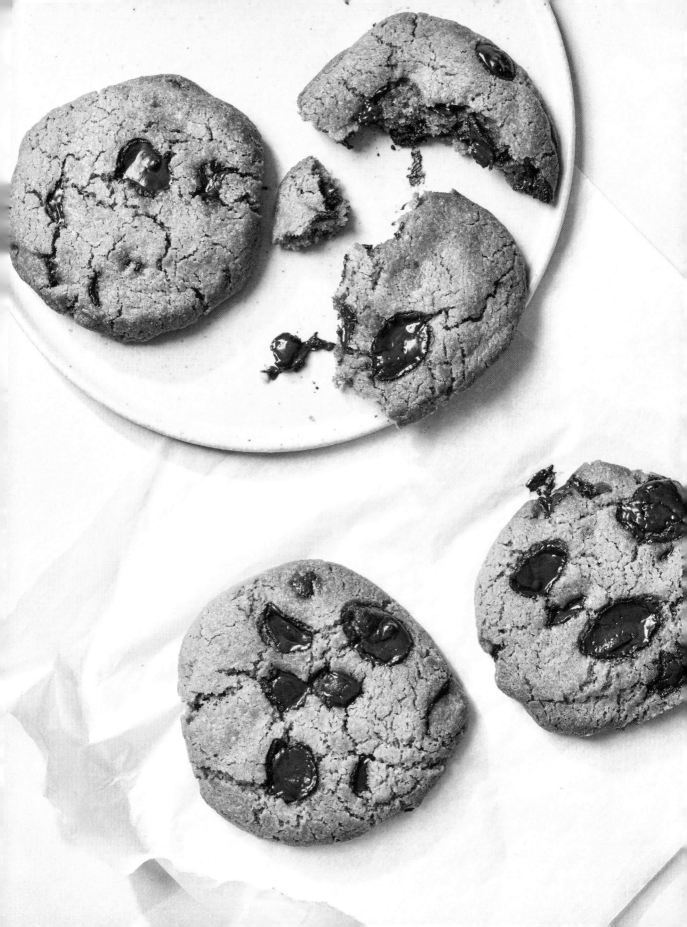

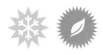

WELSH CAKES

MAKES 25
PREP TIME 20 minutes
COOK TIME 16 minutes

Traditionally, Welsh cakes are made on a griddle, but you can use the air fryer to make your own version of these little lightly spiced flat cakes dotted with sweet currants. They are perfect for sharing with friends over a cup of tea.

115g (4oz) plain flour, plus more to dust

115g (4oz) wholemeal flour

1 teaspoon baking powder

1 teaspoon mixed spice

55g (2oz) butter, cut into small cubes

50g (1¾oz) fat-free Greek yogurt

50g (1¾oz) caster sugar

50g (1¾oz) currants

1 egg, lightly beaten

1 tablespoon (15g / ½oz) honey

2 teaspoons granulated sugar

1   In a mixing bowl, combine the plain and wholemeal flours, baking powder and mixed spice. Add the cubed butter and use your fingers to rub it in and produce a crumb-like consistency, ensuring no big lumps remain. Stir through the yogurt, caster sugar and currants, then work in the egg and honey, using a spatula, to form a soft dough.

2   Bring the dough together into a ball, then lay it on a floured surface and roll it out to about 5mm (¼ inch) thick. Use a 6cm (2½ inch) fluted round cutter to cut out 25 circles.

3   Preheat both air fryer drawers to 180°C (350°F). You will need to cook these in 2 batches, so, once the air fryer has preheated, add 8 Welsh cakes to each drawer (they can go straight on to the crisper plates, but line them with nonstick baking paper if you prefer).

4   Cook for 8 minutes in total, giving them 5 minutes on the first side, then flipping (I use silicone tongs for this) and giving them 3 minutes on the other side. By this time, they should be a lovely golden-brown colour. If they are looking undercooked, give them a couple more minutes. Repeat to cook the second batch.

5   Place the hot Welsh cakes on a plate and sprinkle them with the granulated sugar. These are delicious eaten warm or cold.

PER CAKE

CALORIES	FAT	SAT FAT	CARBS	SUGARS	FIBRE	PROTEIN	SALT
70	2.2G	1.2G	11G	4.5G	0.7G	1.5G	0.11G

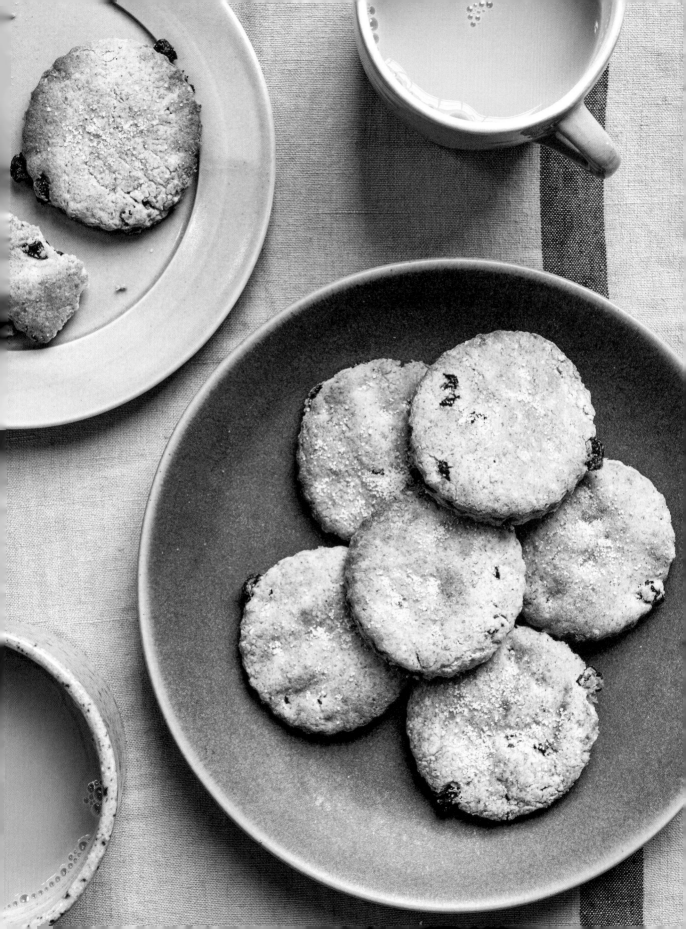

INDEX

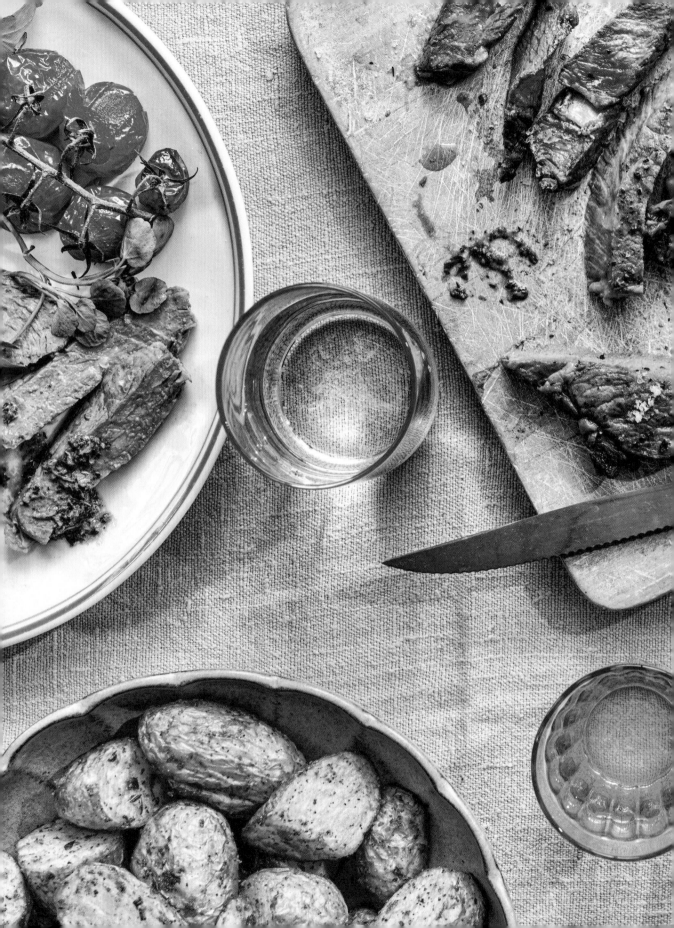

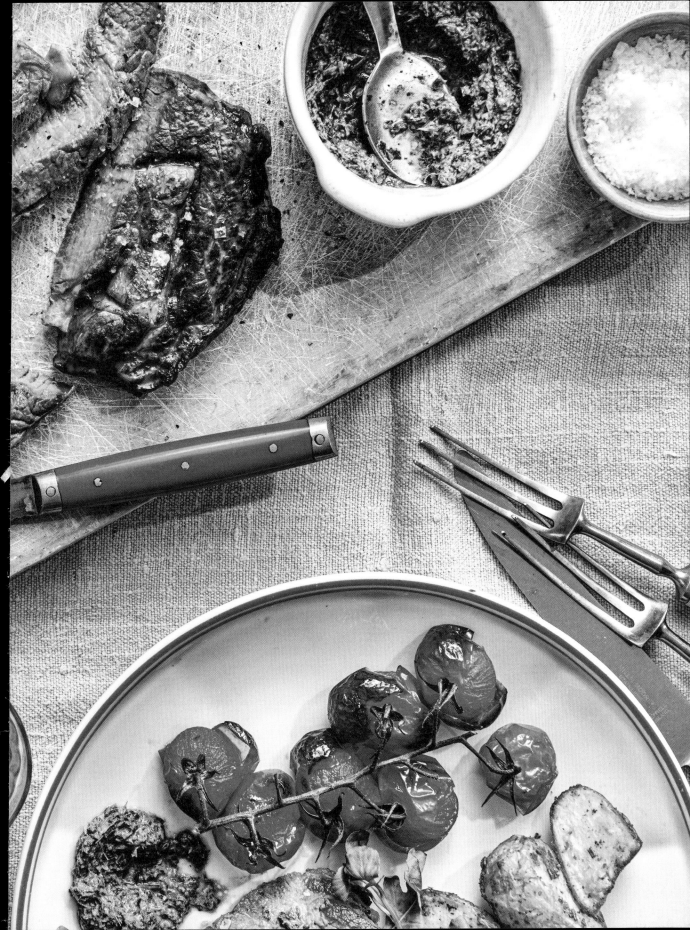

GLOSSARY

UK	US
AUBERGINE	EGGPLANT
BAKING PAPER	PARCHMENT PAPER
BICARBONATE OF SODA	BAKING SODA
BUTTER BEANS	LIMA BEANS
CASTER SUGAR	SUPERFINE SUGAR
CHILLI FLAKES	CRUSHED RED PEPPER
CHIPS	FRIES
CLINGFILM	PLASTIC WRAP
CORIANDER	CILANTRO
CORNFLOUR	CORN STARCH
COURGETTE	ZUCCHINI
DEMERARA SUGAR	TURBINADO SUGAR
GAMMON	FRESH HAM
GOLDEN SYRUP	LIGHT TREACLE
GROUND ALMONDS	ALMOND FLOUR
KITCHEN PAPER	PAPER TOWELS
MARS BAR	MILKY WAY BAR
MINCED MEAT	GROUND MEAT
PLAIN FLOUR	ALL-PURPOSE FLOUR
PORRIDGE OATS	OATMEAL
PRAWNS (KING)	SHRIMP (JUMBO)
PUMPKIN SEEDS	PEPITAS
RED/GREEN PEPPERS	BELL PEPPERS
SEMI-SKIMMED MILK	2 PER CENT MILK
SPRING ONIONS	SCALLIONS
SULTANAS	GOLDEN RAISINS
TEA TOWEL	DISH CLOTH
WHOLEMEAL	WHOLEWHEAT

ACKNOWLEDGEMENTS

I am so incredibly grateful to every single one of you who has supported *The Slimming Foodie* – whether you've been following along on social media, visiting the blog, trying out recipes or buying my cookbooks. Your kind words, photos of your meals and positive interactions keep me motivated every day. I feel very lucky to have such a fantastic and inspiring community – thank you from the bottom of my heart!

There's a brilliant team behind the scenes helping me bring these cookbooks to life, and I couldn't do it without them. A huge thank you to Lucy Bannell for your eagle-eyed attention to detail, making sure everything flows beautifully. I'm also beyond grateful to the team at Octopus. You've made me feel so welcome from the very beginning, and I genuinely couldn't ask for a more supportive and encouraging group to work with. Special shout-outs to Natalie Bradley, Kate Fox, Sybella Stephens, Yasia Williams, Geoff Fennell, Lucy Carter, Nic Jones, Karen Baker and Erin Brown. And thank you to everyone else at Octopus who's played a part in shaping this project.

I'm incredibly fortunate to have worked again with the same dream shoot team who have been at my side for all my previous books: Chris Terry, Tamsin Weston and Henrietta Clancy – you make everything look so stunning, and it's always such fun to work with you. Thanks as well to the wonderful assistant food stylists, Louise Richardson, Natalia Zubenko, Stella Dwyer and Chiara Lancia – your hard work is greatly appreciated.

On a personal note, a massive thank you to my husband Darren, and my two wonderful daughters, Miette and Marlie, for being my constant support team at home. And a big thanks to Sarah and Maria for your tireless work in helping me manage the Facebook group – I am so grateful for all you do!